Gerson Therapy Handbook

Companion workbook to "A Cancer Therapy: Results of Fifty Cases"

Practical guidance, resources, and recipes for following the Gerson Therapy

Revised Fifth Edition

GERSON
INSTITUTE

A non-profit organization dedicated to the holistic treatment of degenerative disease

1572 Second Avenue
San Diego, CA 92101

Tel: (619) 685-5353
Toll Free: 1-888-4-GERSON
Fax: (619) 685-5363

MAIL@GERSON.ORG WWW.GERSON.ORG

Gerson™ Therapy Handbook
Revised Fifth Edition

ISBN: 0-9611526-4-8

A Companion to *A Cancer Therapy: Results of Fifty Cases*, by Max Gerson, M.D.

Table of Contents

Introduction

Throughout our lives our bodies are being filled with a variety of disease and cancer causing pollutants. These toxins reach us through the air we breathe, the food we eat, the medicines we take and the water we drink. As more of these poisons are used every day and cancer rates continue to climb, being able to turn to a proven, natural, detoxifying treatment like the Gerson Therapy is not only reassuring, but necessary.

The Gerson Therapy is a powerful, natural treatment that boosts your body's own immune system to heal cancer, arthritis, heart disease, allergies, and many other degenerative diseases. One aspect of the Gerson Therapy that sets it apart from most other treatment methods is its all-encompassing nature. An abundance of nutrients from thirteen fresh, organic juices are consumed every day, providing your body with a superdose of enzymes, minerals and nutrients. These substances then help the body to break down diseased tissues, while enemas aid in eliminating the lifelong buildup of toxins from the liver.

With its whole-body approach to healing, the Gerson Therapy naturally reactivates your body's magnificent ability to heal itself - with no damaging side-effects. Over 200 articles in respected medical literature, and thousands of people cured of their "incurable" diseases document the Gerson Therapy's effectiveness. The Gerson Therapy is one of the few treatments to have a 60 year history of success.

Although its philosophy of cleansing and reactivating the body is simple, the Gerson Therapy is a complex method of treatment requiring significant attention to detail. While many patients have made full recoveries practicing the Gerson Therapy on their own, for best results, we encourage starting treatment at a Gerson Institute-certified treatment center.

Since the original publication of *A Cancer Therapy: Results of 50 Cases* in 1958, many developments have taken place in the medical world, including the widespread use of (toxic) chemotherapy, the standardization of heart-lung and liver transplants and a rising incidence of cancer in well over a third of our population. At the same time, we have witnessed the emergence of a host of new and often "unexplainable" chronic diseases, such as CFS (Chronic Fatigue Syndrome), lupus (SLE), Legionnaire's disease, AIDS, osteoporosis, and Alzheimer's.

As conventional medicine unearths more clues about the nature of chronic, degenerative disease, evidence has increasingly pointed toward the scientific validity of Dr. Gerson's principles. Virtually all research that has been done in the area of nutrition in the past 50 years has tended to confirm Dr. Gerson's empirical findings. This comes as no surprise to us. Where traditional treatments have failed, we have found that both old and new illnesses alike have proven remarkably susceptible to treatment with the Gerson Therapy.

Whether you intend to beat your "incurable" disease at home or at a Gerson certified clinic, this *Gerson Therapy Handbook* is intended as a user-friendly companion guide to the deservedly more famous but more technical *A Cancer Therapy: Results of 50 Cases*, by Max Gerson, M.D. The latter book contains, in a remarkably condensed form, the accumulated wisdom of 50 years of clinical experimentation in Europe and the United States by Dr. Gerson, who counted heads of state and at least one Nobel laureate among his cured patients. If you plan to undertake the Gerson Therapy we suggest you read both volumes as they work together to provide you with the information you need to begin and maintain the Gerson healing process.

The *Gerson Therapy Handbook* has been organized so that you can find answers quickly and begin the healing process immediately. In the following chapters you will find everything you need to know about the Gerson protocol, from juicing schedules and enema formulas, to the interpretation of lab results. This *Gerson Therapy Handbook* will alert you to crucial healing reactions and it will explain several adjuvant therapies that you may pursue in conjunction with the Gerson Therapy. We have also selected some important articles from issues of the Gerson Healing Newsletter that discuss coffee enemas, pesticides and the merits of organic food in greater detail.

As you face perhaps the greatest challenge of your

life we would like to reassure you that there is both hope and an alternative to the so called cures of traditional medicine. If you have any questions after reading this *Gerson Therapy Handbook* that remain unanswered, please do not hesitate to contact our staff at the Gerson Institute. We wish you well.

The Gerson Institute

The Gerson Institute (a.k.a. Cancer Curing Society) is a non-profit organization dedicated to healing and preventing chronic, degenerative diseases based on the vision, philosophy and the successful work of Dr. Max Gerson.

Founded in 1978 by Charlotte Gerson (daughter of Dr. Gerson) the Gerson Institute provides a range of programs designed to inform and educate the general public and health care practitioners about the benefits of the Gerson Therapy.

Whether you are interested in an alternative treatment for your "incurable" disease, or simply wish to adopt a healthier lifestyle for yourself and your family, the Gerson Institute can help.

Contact our offices by telephone, fax, e-mail or via the internet to find out more about these and other programs that are offered by the Gerson Institute:

Referral to a Licensed Gerson Clinic
Practitioner Training Program
Practitioner Referral List
Care-givers Training Weekend
Gerson Support Groups
Free Brochures
Recovered Patient Referral List
Recovered Patient Support Network
Web Site Chat Rooms
Speaker's Forum
Outreach Program (schools and businesses)
Membership
Subscription to the *Gerson Healing Newsletter*
Advertising & Sponsorship Opportunities
Calendar of Events
National & International Seminars and Workshops
The Tree of Life
Books & Tapes
Library Donation Program

* Programs will change from time to time. Please contact the Gerson Institute for current information.

Mailing address:

1572 Second Avenue
San Diego, CA 92101

Telephone: (619) 685-5353
Fax: (619) 685-5363
Toll Free: 1-888-4-GERSON

Please Note: *The Gerson Institute does not own, operate, or control any treatment facility. We maintain a licensing program with clinics to ensure that patients are receiving true, 100% Gerson care. Be sure your clinic is Gerson Institute Certified to provide the Gerson Therapy. Phone the Gerson Institute to discuss how the Gerson Therapy can help you.*

We will be happy to answer your questions: 1-888-4-GERSON.

Max Gerson, M.D. and the Gerson Therapy

Max Gerson, M.D. was born October 18, 1881 in Wongrowitz, Germany. He attended the universities of Breslau, Wuerzburg and Berlin, eventually graduating from the University of Freiburg. Suffering from severe migraines, Dr. Max Gerson focused his initial dietary experiments on preventing these debilitating headaches. It was discovered in the course of treatment with this special "migraine diet", that one of Dr. Gerson's patients was cured of his skin tuberculosis. This discovery led to further studies of the diet, and to Dr. Gerson successfully treating many more tuberculosis patients.

After some time, his work came to the attention of famed thoracic surgeon, Ferdinand Sauerbruch, M.D. With the help and supervision of Dr. Sauerbruch, Gerson established a skin tuberculosis treatment program at the Munich University Hospital. In a carefully monitored clinical trial, 446 out of 450 skin tuberculosis patients treated with Gerson's dietary regimen, experienced complete recoveries. Dr. Sauerbruch and Dr. Gerson simultaneously published articles on the study in a dozen of the world's leading medical journals, establishing the Gerson treatment as the first cure for skin tuberculosis.

Through his work with tuberculosis, Dr. Gerson attracted the friendship of Nobel Peace Prize recipient, Albert Schweitzer, M.D. At the time, Dr. Schweitzer's interest in Gerson was prompted by conventional methods having failed to cure his wife, Helene Schweitzer-Bresslau (1879-1957), of lung tuberculosis. In 1930, after suffering her tuberculosis for seven years, Helene was admitted to Dr. Gerson's clinic and cured after 9 months. The two doctors shared a good friendship for the rest of their lives. It came to pass that even Schweitzer's own advanced (Type II) diabetes was cured by Gerson's nutritional therapy. Schweitzer followed Gerson's progress over the years, seeing the dietary therapy successfully applied further to heart disease, kidney failure, and then finally - cancer.

To escape Adolf Hitler's reign in Europe, Dr. Gerson moved with his family to America, where they took up residence in New York. In 1938, Dr. Gerson passed his medical boards and was then licensed to practice medicine in the state of New York. For twenty years, he treated hundreds of cancer patients who had been given up to die after all conventional treatments had failed. In 1946, Dr. Gerson demonstrated some of these recovered patients before the Pepper-Neely Congressional Subcommittee. The committee was holding hearings on a bill to fund research into cancer treatment. Although only a handful of peer-reviewed journals were receptive to Gerson's then "radical" idea of diet affecting health, he continued publishing articles on his therapy in Europe and presenting case histories of his healed patients. In 1958, after thirty years of clinical experimentation, Gerson published *A Cancer Therapy: Results of Fifty Cases.* This medical monograph details the theories, treatment, and results achieved by a great physician. In 1959 Dr. Max Gerson died.

It was 50 years ago that Dr. Gerson promoted better health through nutrition. Although ridiculed in his time, today, we are shown proof in countless articles and studies, that he was merely ahead of his time. As better diet proves to be the answer to healing more and more of our health problems, the words of Dr. Gerson's good friend carry a deeply prophetic ring.

"I see in him one of the most eminent geniuses in the history of medicine. Many of his basic ideas have been adopted without having his name connected with them. Yet, he has achieved more than seemed possible under adverse conditions. He leaves a legacy which commands attention and which will assure him his due place. Those whom he has cured will now attest to the truth of his ideas."

- Nobel Prize Laureate and healed Gerson patient, Dr. Albert Schweitzer, in eulogy of Max Gerson, M.D.

The Gerson Therapy

The Gerson Therapy is a state of the art, contemporary, holistic and natural treatment which utilizes the body's own healing mechanism in the treatment and cure of chronic debilitating illness. When it was introduced to the world by Max Gerson, M.D., the dietary therapy was so far ahead of its time that there were almost no rationales available in the scientific literature to explain how it could produce cures in chronic as well as infectious diseases. But, because it did cure many cases of advanced tuberculosis, heart disease, cancer and numerous lesser conditions, the Gerson Therapy was established as a major contribution to the medical field, through the publication of hundreds of articles in peer reviewed medical literature. Gerson first published on the topic of cancer in 1945, almost forty years before the adoption of the current official U.S. National Cancer Institute program on diet, nutrition, and cancer. Today, leaders in the medical establishment predict a 50% reduction in cancers by the year 2000 through educating the public in dietary methods of preventing cancer.

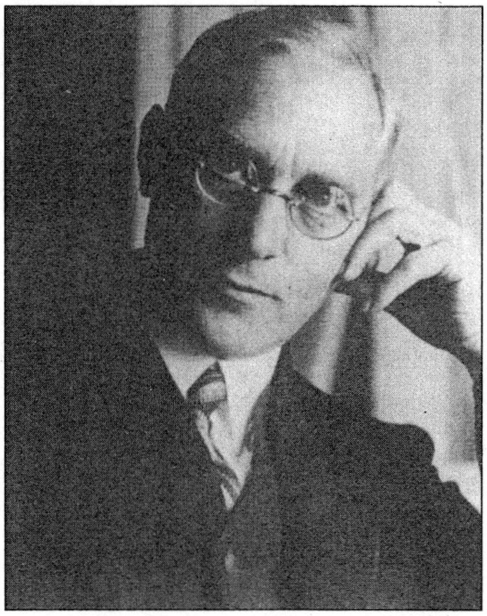

Max Gerson, M.D. (1881-1959)

It is rare to find cancer, arthritis, or other degenerative diseases in cultures considered "primitive" by Western civilization. Is it because of diet? The fact that degenerative diseases appear in these cultures only when modern packaged foods and additives are introduced would certainly support that idea. Max Gerson said "Stay close to nature and its eternal laws will protect you." He considered that degenerative diseases were brought on by toxic, degraded food, water and air.

The Gerson Therapy seeks to regenerate the body to health, supporting each important metabolic requirement by flooding the body with nutrients from almost 20 pounds of organically grown fruits and vegetables daily. Most is used to make fresh raw juice, one glass every hour, 13 times per day. Raw and cooked solid foods are generously consumed. Oxygenation is usually more than doubled, as oxygen deficiency in the blood contributes to many degenerative diseases. The metabolism is also stimulated through the addition of thyroid, potassium and other supplements, and by avoiding heavy animal fats, excess protein, sodium and other toxins.

Degenerative diseases render the body increasingly unable to excrete waste materials adequately, commonly resulting in liver and kidney failure. To prevent this, the Gerson Therapy uses intensive detoxification to eliminate wastes, regenerate the liver, reactivate the immune system and restore the body's essential defenses - enzyme, mineral and hormone systems. With generous, high-quality nutrition, increased oxygen availability, detoxification, and improved metabolism, the cells - and the body - can regenerate, become healthy and prevent future illness.

Dr. Patricia Spain Ward, *History of the Gerson Therapy*, 1988

It is one of the least edifying facts of recent American medical history that the profession's leadership so long neglected as quackish the idea that nutrition affects health (*JAMA* 1946, 1949, 1977; Shimkin, 1976). Ignoring both the empirical dietary wisdom that pervaded western medicine from the pre-Christian Hippocratic era until the late nineteenth century and a persuasive body of modern research in nutritional biochemistry, the politically minded spokesmen of organized medicine in the U.S. remained long committed to surgery and radiation as the sole acceptable treatments for cancer. This commitment persisted, even after sound epidemiological data showed that early detection and removal of malignant tumors did not "cure" most kinds of cancer (Crile, 1956; updated by Cairns, 1985).

The historical record shows that progress lagged especially in cancer immunotherapy – including nutrition and hyperthermia - because power over professional affiliation and publication (and hence over practice and research) rested with men who were neither scholars nor practitioners nor researchers themselves, and who were often unequipped to grasp the rapidly evolving complexities of the sciences underlying mid-twentieth century medicine.

Nowhere is this maladaptation of professional structure to medicine's changing scientific content more tragically illustrated than in the American experience of Max B. Gerson (1881-1959), founder of the best-known nutritional treatment for cancer of the pre-macrobiotic era. A scholar's scholar and a superlative observer of clinical phenomena, Gerson was a product of the German medical education which Americans in the late 19th and early 20th centuries considered so superior to our own that all who could afford it went to Germany to perfect their training (Bonnier, 1963).

As a medical graduate of the University of Freiburg in 1909, Gerson imbibed all of the latest in scientific medicine, with the emphasis on specificity which bacteriology had brought into Western medical thought in the preceding decades. Gerson subsequently worked with leading German specialists in internal medicine, in physiological chemistry, and in neurology (U.S. Congress, 1946, 98). The historical record does not tell us whether his medical education in Germany (where much of the early work in nutritional chemistry took place) included a study of diet, a subject neglected in American medical schools after the germ theory gained acceptance.

We do know that by 1919, when Gerson set up a practice in internal and nervous diseases in Bielefeld, he had devised an effective dietary treatment for the migraine headaches which frequently disabled him, despite the best efforts of his colleagues. In 1920, while treating migraine patients by this salt-free vegetarian diet, he discovered that it was also effective in lupus vulgaris (tuberculosis at the skin, then considered incurable) and, later, in arthritis as well (U.S. Congress, 1946, 98).

Trained in the theories of specific disease causation and treatment that began to dominate western medicine for the first time in history - as bacteriological discoveries multiplied in the late nineteenth century, Gerson was at first uneasy about using a single therapy in such seemingly disparate conditions. But he was committed to the primacy of clinical evidence, which he liked to express in Kussmaul's dictum: "The result at the sick-bed is decisive" (quoted in Gerson, 1958, 212).

- Dr. Patricia Spain Ward, *History of the Gerson Therapy*, 1988.

Wishing you good health,
Gerson Institute

Chapter 1: Procedures Used While in the Hospital

> Before attempting your first enema please request assistance from your duty nurse or Gerson doctor.

Enemas

Getting started

Following admission, under physicians orders, you should have been issued:

- Plastic enema bucket with plastic hose
- Jar of coffee
- Distilled water dispenser
- Pad to place under you while taking enemas
- Vaseline
- Hotplate

Coffee Enemas

(Reference: *A Cancer Therapy: Results of Fifty Cases*, pp. 190, 247). Timing and frequency of enemas will vary throughout the entirety of your therapy. Your physician will instruct you and answer questions concerning use of coffee enemas.

Helpful Hints:

- Always keep the pot with the distilled water on the warmer. It will not boil and will always be ready.
- If your bucket's plastic hose becomes kinked, run a small amount of hot water through it to soften it.

General Procedure for Coffee Enemas

The coffee solution should be used at body temperature. Run a little of the solution through the tube into the toilet to warm the tube and get rid of the air; close the stopcock. Lubricate rectal or enema tube for about 2" at end with petroleum jelly. Hang the enema bucket not more than two feet above you. Lying on your right side, draw both legs close to the abdomen, relax and breathe deeply.

Insert the tube into your rectum 5" to 8". Open the stopcock and allow fluid to run in very slowly to avoid cramping. Retain the solution for 12-15 minutes.

If you have trouble retaining or taking in the full 32 oz., lower the bucket; if you feel spasms, lower the bucket to the floor to allow the flow to back up a bit to relieve the pressure. After 12-20 seconds, slowly start raising the bucket toward its original level. You can also control the flow of solution by pinching the tube with your fingers or adjusting the plastic ring in a partially closed position. You will quickly learn what works best for you.

Keep your equipment clean!

Don't place the tube back into the bucket until after you have thoroughly cleaned both the tube and the bucket. Use a biodegradable, food-use detergent and/or hydrogen peroxide and rinse well. Rinse at least once a day with hydrogen peroxide 3%. The bucket and the tube are very good growing grounds for bacteria.

Frequency of Enemas

Frequency of enemas is increased with symptoms of toxicity such as headache, fever, nausea, intestinal spasms and drowsiness. Upon awakening in the morning if headache and drowsiness are experienced, an additional enema is recommended during the following night.

Nourish first - then detoxify.

As a general rule, eat some raw or steamed fruit before

Good Ideas!

Vital sign records

It is important to learn to keep records of your own vital signs (temperature and pulse). Your pulse and temperature should be taken daily before you get out of bed and move about. Keep the thermometer right next to your bed. If your pulse should near 120/min, the thyroid dosage may need to be reduced. An increase in temperature can be a sign of an impending "flare-up."

Keep food in your room

- A fruit plate is delivered to your room daily. Please ask for more if you need it.
- Keep thermoses of hot peppermint tea prepared (especially at night).
- Don't drink water that may compete with the juices.
- Have enough coffee in your room to take enemas during the night and in the early morning before breakfast.

your first coffee enema of the day to activate the upper digestive tract. A small piece of fruit is sufficient. This rule applies whenever considerable time has elapsed since the last meal, juice or snack.

Castor Oil Treatment

Castor oil by mouth

(Reference: *A Cancer Therapy: Results of Fifty Cases*, pp. 81, 247). Every other day, 2 tablespoons of castor oil are given by mouth at about 5:30 AM, followed by a cup of black coffee with raw brown sugar. The coffee serves to stimulate the musculature of the stomach to empty the castor oil into the small intestine, thus lessening the discomfort of the castor oil.

To avoid stuffiness and cramping with castor oil by mouth, eat frequently and drink peppermint tea. **Please see footnote 19, pp. 247-248, *A Cancer Therapy - Results of 50 Cases.***

Castor oil enema

(Reference: *A Cancer Therapy: Results of Fifty Cases*, pp. 191, 247). At about 10:30 AM, 5 hours after your castor oil by mouth, the castor oil enema will be brought to your room to be administered. The castor oil should be mixed first with 1/2 tsp. Ox-bile powder, then with the coffee for optimum results. Because oil and water normally separate, you need to swish a bar of soap (not detergent "bar") around briefly in the coffee to help the two liquids mix. Be careful not to get too much soap into the coffee, since soap can irritate the colon. Add the castor oil to the solution, and stir. The solution should be stirred continuously during the enema, since the oil will still tend to separate from the coffee. If you are not a contortionist, have somebody stir the solution for you. You may retain the castor oil enema for a short time, but it is not required.

Medications

(Reference: *A Cancer Therapy: Results of Fifty Cases*, pp. 235,236,236b). Each morning, the nursing staff will supply you with your daily medications in a plastic box divided into compartments marked with the hour of the day each pill is to be taken.

Please return your medication box to a nurse after dinner. It will be refilled and returned to you.

Mealtime medications

- Acidol pepsin - before each meal.
- Pancreatin tablets - when the meal is completed.
- Other medications - during the meal.

Time	Juices 8 oz. each	Diet	Medication: Linseed oil, Tbsp. p.246	Acidol Pepsin, Caps	Potassium Compound Solution, tsp. in juice	Lugol 1/2 stregnth, drops in juice	Thyroid 1 gr. tablet	Niacin 50 mg. tablet	Pancreatin, tablet	Royal Jelly 50 mg. caps.	Injection, 100 mcg B-12 combined with 3cc liver	Coffee Enemas	Castor Oil Treatment	Tests
8:00	Orange	Breakfast		2	4	3	1	1	3		Once Daily	Every 4 Hours	Every Other Day	As Directed
9:00	Green				4									
9:30	Apple-Carrot				4	3								
10:00	Apple-Carrot				4	3	1	1						
11:00	Carrot													
12:00	Green	2 Liver Capsules			4									
1:00	Apple-Carrot	Lunch	1	2	4	3	1	1	3					
2:00	Green				4									
3:00	Carrot													
4:00	Carrot	2 Liver Capsules												
5:00	Apple-Carrot	2 Liver Capsules			4	3	1	1	3					
6:00	Green				4			1						
7:00	Apple-Carrot	Dinner	1	2	4	3	1	1	3					

Annotated hourly schedule

(Written for the 3rd edition of *A Cancer Therapy - Results of 50 Cases*.) Patients and assistants should read and understand pages 187-248 and Appendix II of *A Cancer Therapy: Results of Fifty Cases* before attempting to reproduce the treatment at home.

> **CAUTION:** The above schedule reflects normal diet and dosages for the initial weeks of treatment. As suggested by the following note, it is essential that the diet and dosages be regularly adjusted by a physician trained in the Gerson Therapy.

Call your Gerson consulting physician to discuss adjustments to your schedule.

Diet and Juices:

The diet and juices are described on **pp. 187-190, 235, and 237-245 of *A Cancer Therapy: Results of Fifty Cases***. The diet must be modified during reactions and flare-ups **(pp. 190, 201-203 of *A Cancer Therapy: Results of Fifty Cases*)**. Soured, nonfat dairy proteins (yogurt and unsalted, non-fat pot cheese) should be added at (not before) the 6th to 8th week according to the physician's judgement **(pp. 80, 145, 146, 235 of *A Cancer Therapy: Results of Fifty Cases*)**.

Exceptions: use churned, not cultured buttermilk. Because low nutrient levels and pesticide content of commercial produce may prevent healing, organically grown produce is extremely important **(pp. 146-151, 167-185, 220, 410 of *A Cancer Therapy: Results of Fifty Cases*)**.

Flax Seed Oil (a.k.a. Linseed Oil):

Never fry, cook, or heat oil. Cold pressed flax seed oil plays an important role in the therapy and should be included. Cold pressed oil must be used because heating changes chemical composition, making it damaging to the body. Linseed oil assists the body in utilizing Vitamin A, a fat soluble vitamin. It is a source of linoleic acid, as well as lacking in cholesterol and effective in lowering cholesterol in the blood. During the first month of therapy, two tablespoons of flaxseed oil per day are given. Following the first month and during the balance of the therapy the use is limited to one tablespoon per day. Follow your physician's orders. For more detailed information, see the ***Gerson Healing Newsletter*, No. 22-23, 1988: "Fats that Heal, Fats that Kill."**

Acidol Pepsin:

capsules are the source of supplemental hydrochloric acid and pepsin, a digestive enzyme, used by Dr. Gerson. Take BEFORE meal.

Potassium:

(10% solution, **see pg. 246 of *A Cancer Therapy: Results of Fifty Cases***) - Dosage (first 3-4 weeks): 4 tsp. solution in each of 10 orange, carrot/apple, and green-juices (10x4 tsp. daily). Thereafter. the physician will normally reduce the dosage to 10x2 tsp. for 20 weeks, then 8x2 for 12 weeks, and 6x2 for the duration of treatment. However, more frequent adjustments by the physician are common **(pp.207-208, 235, 246, 393, 409, 410 of *A Cancer Therapy: Results of Fifty Cases*)**. When you arrive home, place one 100 gm. container of potassium compound salts into a one quart glass jar and fill to the top with distilled water. Store bottle in a dark place. Does not need refrigeration.

Lugol's Solution:

(half-strength) Dosage (first 3-4 weeks only): 3 drops in each of 6 orange and carrot/apple juices (6x3 daily). **Do not put Lugol's in green juice.** Thereafter, the physician will normally reduce the dosage to 6x1 for 8 weeks, and 3x1 for the duration of treatment. Lugol's solution is a 10% solution of 10 gm. potassium iodide and 5 gm. iodine in water to total 100 ml. of solute. The Lugol's Solution for Gerson patients is premixed half strength (5% solution). Use Lugol's as supplied. Do not dilute **(pp. 32, 205, 235, 246, 409 of *A Cancer Therapy: Results of Fifty Cases*)**.

Thyroid:

Dosage (first 3-4 weeks only): 5x1 grain daily. In the example case on **page 235 of *A Cancer Therapy: Results of Fifty Cases***, the dosage was reduced to 3x1/2 grain for 8 weeks, then 3x1/4 grain for 14 weeks. More frequent adjustments by the physician are common. Tachycardia (pulse over 120) may indicate overdosage. Discontinue temporarily during menses **(pp. 205, 206, 235, 246, 409 of *A Cancer Therapy: Results of Fifty Cases*)**.

Niacin:

Dosage: 50 mg at least 6 times daily for 6 months. In advanced cases, Dr. Gerson used 50 mg. every hour around the clock (Rev. Gastroenterol, 12(6):419, 1945). Reactions (flushing: hot, red skin) are temporary and harmless. Minor bleedings are no cause for concern, but discontinue during menses or in case of hemorrhage. Niacinamide is not allowed. Use only niacin **(pp. 99, 209,235,246 of *A Cancer Therapy: Results of Fifty Cases*)**.

Pancreatin:

Dosage: 3 tablets 4 times daily, or according to patient's needs. A few patients do not tolerate pancreatin well, but most benefit with less digestive trouble, gas spasms, and less difficulty gaining weight and strength **(pp. 211, 212, 235, 246, 411 of *A Cancer Therapy: Results of Fifty Cases*)**.

Royal Jelly:

(optional) - Dosage: 100 mg. in capsules or honey, one hour before breakfast. Do not take with hot food. Available from some health food stores **(pp. 200, 235 of *A Cancer Therapy: Results of Fifty Cases*)**.

Liver Extract (crude) and B_{12}:

(by injection): Dosage: 3 cc liver and 0.1 cc B_{12} combined in a single syringe, injected into gluteus medius daily, for 4-6 months or more. The physician will normally reduce frequency gradually over the course of therapy **(pp. 80-82, 196, 210-211, 235, 240, 246, 393, 407, 409, 411, 412 of *A Cancer Therapy: Results of Fifty Cases*)**.

Coffee Enemas:

(pg. 247 of *A Cancer Therapy: Results of Fifty Cases*) - Dosage (first 6 weeks minimum): While lying on right side, retain for 12-15 minutes - EVERY FOUR HOURS. For limited periods of time, against severe pain, coffee enemas may be used as frequently as every two hours. However, physician must monitor serum electrolytes frequently.

Castor oil:

Dosage: 2 Tbsp. by mouth and five hours later a castor oil and soap enema **(pg. 247 of *A Cancer Therapy: Results of Fifty Cases*)** EVERY OTHER DAY. Later, as necessary or as prescribed, **(pp. 81, 166, 190-195, 198, 201-203. 206. 235, 393, 406-410, 416-418 of *A Cancer Therapy: Results of Fifty Cases*)**.

Tests:

Blood Chemistry, Complete Blood Count, T3, T4, Urinalysis - All tests should be taken before beginning treatment and at 4-6 week intervals for at least the first 6 months. Test results may be affected by healing reactions and flare-ups **(pp. 235, 415 of *A Cancer Therapy: Results of Fifty Cases*)**. ***(See Appendix I: Lab Tests, for a more in depth description of tests, Pg. 33)***. ***Note:*** *Please mail or fax copies of all blood work to your Gerson consulting physician.*

All other Medications:

Do not abruptly discontinue any medications you are taking prior to using the Gerson Therapy. In certain cases, Gerson trained physicians will advise gradual discontinuance.

Vitamin C (Ascorbic Acid)

This substance is employed in the Gerson Therapy during infections. A crystalline (powdered) form such as Bronson's is preferred. The Gerson diet contains large amounts of natural Vitamin C, so routine daily supplementation should not be necessary.

Bee pollen:

This is an addition to the Gerson program that can be employed in cancer from about the tenth to twelfth week. Non-cancer patients can start earlier, about the sixth week. Some patients may have allergies to bee pollen. The initial dosage is 1/2 tsp. per day.

Liver juice:

Liver Juice has been discontinued. Substitute: Carrot juice plus 2 liver capsules for each liver juice. **(Reference, A Cancer Therapy: Results of Fifty Cases, Appendix III, pg. 421)**

Adjuvant Therapies

Because the Gerson Therapy is your primary management, any agent, material, technique, or procedure added to the Gerson Therapy must be characterized as adjuvant, or supportive in nature, e.g.: when a Gerson patient elects to use laetrile, the new material cannot replace the central and continuous work of the Gerson Therapy. The Gerson Therapy must not be altered in the hope of improving the performance of the laetrile (some laetrile therapists recommend dietary measures which would be counter-productive if introduced into the Gerson Therapy). Always consult your Gerson Therapy Physician with regard to ANY promising new addition to your treatment.

The following procedures and materials are among those that are available at Gerson facilities in a form compatible with the Gerson Therapy. It is important to remember that each Gerson Therapy Center is separately owned and operated under the certification guidelines of the Gerson Institute. The following or additional therapies may be available at any given facility. Your Gerson physician may choose to recommend the addition of one or more additional procedures to your therapy.

Amygdalin/Laetrile:

Laetrile is the purified form of amygdalin, also called vitamin B-17, which occurs naturally in the pits of apricots and in some other foods. Laetrile is a cyanogenic glycoside (containing cyanide). While we believe laetrile to be non-toxic, laetrile by itself does not cure. It has been used at some Gerson Therapy facilities as an analgesic (for pain relief). Laetrile has other purported anti-cancer properties. Gerson patients may request laetrile from their physician, but it is not part of the routine Gerson Therapy.

Polarizing Treatment:

One addition to the Gerson therapy protocol is the polarizing treatment pioneered by Dr. Demetrio Sodi-Pallares, a noted Mexico City cardiologist and researcher. He was formerly director of the Mexican Medical Association and the National Institute of Cardiology of Mexico City. He is the author of several books and many articles on cardiology. He places nutrition in its proper role for prevention and treatment of disease.

The basic Polarizing solution (GKI) can be found in *Merck's Manual of Standard Medical Procedures*, a standard medical text. Sodi-Pallares found that in many patients who are deficient in potassium, it is necessary to provide a transport mechanism to help potassium travel through the cell membrane. He achieved this by using a potassium solution (K) together with glucose (G) and a tiny bit of insulin (I) which is given together intravenously.

Polarizing treatment promotes healing in the diseased heart, and in tissues damaged by cancer and other degenerative diseases. Patients with edema (excess fluids in feet, abdomen) note a rapid reabsorption and release of the fluids from the body.

Oxygen therapy:

Preliminary clinical studies indicate that oxidative therapy might produce desirable results in cancer treatment. Most hostile micro-organisms probably require lower oxygen levels than the body's cells. Boosting serum oxygen levels may revitalize normal cells while damaging some viruses and other pathogens. Two basic types of oxygen therapy are ozone therapy and the absorption of hydrogen peroxide at very low concentrations. Hydrogen peroxide (H_2O_2), is produced when ozone (O_3) contacts water. It can be taken orally if diluted with water (1/2% or less), absorbed through the skin by bathing in it (from 4-5 pints of 3% H_2O_2 in a standard size bathtub), used topically, or taken rectally. Ambient air ozone generators are used to benefit patients. In addition to the intensive Gerson Therapy, some adjuvant procedures are being made available to patients. These are scientifically based additions to the Gerson Therapy to add to the patients' ability to heal. Patients should discuss these additions to their treatment with their Gerson physician. Also extra charges will apply, consequently please check with the hospital office.

Adjuvant Treatments

There is much evidence that increasing the patient's blood oxygen level helps fight tumor tissue and increases the body's immune system response.

Phagocytic leukocytes (white blood corpuscles) are the first and most important line of defense against infection. In the daily care of patients, physicians and surgeons usually assume that granulocyte function is normal - unless they have evidence to the contrary. However, data now clearly show that the killing capacity of granulocytes is normal only to the degree to which oxygen is available to them. This is probably the basis for the age-old observation that local immunity is proportional to blood supply.

Normally, leukocytes move and digest bacteria equally well by using anaerobically or aerobically derived energy. However, the capacity of leukocytes to kill bacteria depends largely on molecular oxygen. Bacterial killing is usually conceived of as comprising two major components. The first involves degranulation and ingestion of the bacteria. The second mechanism, called "oxidative killing," depends on molecular oxygen, which is captured by leukocytes and converted to high-energy radicals - such as superoxide, hydroxyl radicals, peroxides, aldehydes, hypochlorite and hypoiodite - which are toxic to bacteria in varying degrees. The rate of production of toxic radicals - and hence the adequacy of oxidative bacterial killing - is directly proportional to local oxygen tension.

The following organisms have been found directly susceptible to oxidative killing:

Staph aureus	Hohn, Surg Forum, 1976
Proteus vulgaris	Mandel G., Infec Immun, 1974
Salmonella typhimurium	Mandel G., Infec Immun, 1974
Klebsiella pneumonia	Mandel G., Infec Immun, 1974
Serratia marcescens	Mandel G., Infec Immun, 1974
Staph albus	McRipley RJ, J Bact, 1967
Pseudomonas aeruginosa	McRipley RJ, J Bact, 1967
Escherichα coli	Selveraj NJ, Nature, 1960

Conclusions:

- Well-oxygenated leukocytes are far more efficient than hypoxic leukocytes.
- Clinically, sufficient hypoxia can occur to inhibit leukocytes and sufficient hyperoxia can easily be achieved to facilitate WBC function.
- The immunological benefits of raising tissue pH; out of the "critical zone" is roughly equivalent to the effects of antibiotics.
- The effects of oxygen and antibiotics are equivalent.

These experiments show that oxygen effects are not only clinically evident, but are clinically important. (The above was taken from the notes of the Winter Symposium on Baromedicine, January 12-15, 1994, by Robert Bartlett, MD, FACEP).

Ozone:

another form of oxygen, is offered by rectal insufflation. About 30cc of ozone is inserted into the rectum from where it is easily absorbed into the blood stream. Ozone is not well tolerated by tumor tissue, while normal tissue is supported by extra oxygen.

Laetrile (amygdalin):

Another treatment which has been used for a number of years is Laetrile. This material is present in as many as 2,400 common foods, grains and grasses. For medicinal purposes, it is extracted mainly from apricot pits. It contains a fraction which helps the body to destroy tumor tissue but is harmless to normal cells. It has been shown that Laetrile, when given to cancer patients, increases the temperature around the tumor - part of its capability of fighting cancer.

Hydrotherapy:

For this treatment, the patient is immersed in a bathtub containing water above body temperature. This will cause a mild induced fever. When Laetrile has already been injected prior to the bath, the temperature at the tumor site is further increased which gives the body a still better opportunity to destroy the tumor tissue. Normal healthy body tissue can easily withstand temperatures up to 104° F, however tumor tissue cannot.

Vitamin C:

Vitamin C is another addition to the adjunctive treatment protocols. It has numerous beneficial effects. It can be used orally and rectally. One protocol uses Laetrile and Vitamin C for the treatment of patients that have previously had chemotherapy.

Wobe Mugos:

These are highly concentrated pancreatic enzymes. The basic Gerson Therapy contains a fair amount of pancreatin. This helps to dissolve and digest tumor tissue. In some patients, especially if they carry a heavy tumor load, the additional intensive pancreatin (Wobe-Mugos) has improved the patient's ability to digest and destroy tumor tissue.

Tahebo Tea (also known as Pau d'Arco) and Essiac Tea:

These are certain herb combinations which have been used by native Indians of the Americas and have been shown to have anti-cancer properties. These teas may be available at your Gerson hospital.

Live Cell Therapy:

This therapy is much more effective after good detoxification and should not be tried during the initial stages of Gerson Therapy. It may be available on request from your Gerson Therapy facility.

Adjuvant Therapeutic Procedures

Pain Relief

Pain medications are often toxic and may interfere with the Gerson diet therapy. Whenever possible, use non-toxic methods to reduce and control pain.

More frequent enemas:

During reactions, pain can be caused or worsened when substantial amounts of toxins are circulating throughout the blood system. They irritate the nerves in damaged and diseased areas of the body. By lowering toxic levels, this irritation and pain can be lessened. This is done by more frequent enemas.

Research has shown that the body has its own natural pain killers. It is thought that some factor in the coffee enema may stimulate the release of these pain killers. Most patients can testify to the fact that enemas relate directly to lowered pain levels.

Pain triad:

The triad should be used sparingly. Do not exceed 6 dosages in a 24 hour period unless prescribed by your physician.

- 50 mg. Niacin
- 500 mg. Ascorbic Acid
- 5 gr. Aspirin

The Pain triad becomes progressively more effective as the body undergoes detoxification. It can be used at bedtime to assist in going to sleep for those patients with substantial pain.

Castor oil pack:

1. Soak 3 pieces of white flannel with castor oil - squeeze out excess castor oil.
2. Place flannel pack over liver or other affected area.
3. Place slightly larger sheet of plastic over the flannel.
4. Use medium temperature heating pad over area. Don't let the pack get cold or uncomfortably hot.
5. Keep on 1-1/2 hours; apply every four hours. You can re-use the castor oil pack.

The castor oil pack is used during severe flare-ups involving liver pain, bile system spasms, or severe pain at other sites. This procedure can also be used by arthritic patients over swollen, painful joints. It is a bit messy when used over hands and feet, but effective.

Hydrotherapy

Hydrotherapy (hot tub bath, hot fomentation) is one of the best remedies for pain. It dulls and calms the pain. Hydrotherapy is also a great assist to detoxification by improving the circulation of the blood and lymphatics. ***Patients with nervous system disease such as MS should not be subjected to high temperature. Cool compresses are more beneficial for these patients.***

The Theory Behind Hydrotherapy

Hydrotherapy may be defined as the use of water in any of its three forms, solid, liquid, or vapor, internally or externally, in the treatment of disease or trauma. Hyperthermia is the application of heat, hot tub bath, hot fomentations, hot foot baths, etc.

Heat treatments play an important role as an adjunct to the Gerson program. Treatments increase heart rate and respiratory rate, increase metabolism important for healing, and increase perspiration which assists in detoxification. Treatments stimulate an increase in leukocytes (white blood cells) and neutrophils, thus mobilizing the body's defenses against disease. The resultant increased blood flow brings about greatly improved oxygenation necessary for proper healing. Oxygenation assists in the fight against cancer which does not like an oxygenated environment. Congestion of internal organs, such as the liver, gall bladder, kidneys, etc., is relieved. Poor circulation is improved. Heat often assists in pain relief. Increased circulation lowers toxin levels thereby reducing the nerve irritation which causes pain. Treatments aid in repair of diseased tissues. They affect not only the immediate skin areas, but also exert reflex effects elsewhere in the body through the nervous system. For instance, heat over the abdominal wall decreases spasms of the intestinal tract; heat over kidneys and lower abdomen increases urine production.

The treatments are non-toxic and safe. Contraindications may be seen in patients with multiple sclerosis (cold hydrotherapy is more beneficial), diabetes, high blood pressure, heart and vascular diseases. These patients will need prior medical review.

For the cancer patient there is an additional important benefit in the hot water treatments. Many types of cancer cells are much more sensitive to heat than are normal cells. If temperatures can be raised high enough (104° F or more) and long enough, death of cancer cells may result. Research has shown that following intravenous or rectal application of laetrile there may be a temperature increase in the tumor mass of 4°-5° F. When this localized increase is added to total body hyperthermia many benefits have been noted, including tumor shrinkage and stimulation of detoxification.

Keep records of all procedures, including date, time, and reactions:

- Hyperthermia treatment
- Hot tub bath
- Procedure

Full treatments should not be taken during healing reactions, though relaxing baths at lower temperatures are allowed. Patients will need to have a medical examination and EKG in preparation. The accompanying person is invited to attend the treatments to observe the procedures so they can be continued in the home environment. ***Do not use chlorinated water for this treatment.***

Preparing for and Undergoing Hydrotherapy

1. Don't eat: Patient should eat nothing for 3-4 hours before treatment. Liquids (juices, tea, etc.) can be continued. If the patient is scheduled soon after a meal, only a light meal may be taken.

2. Coffee enema: One hour before scheduled treatment a coffee enema is taken.

3. Shower: At this time a thorough cleansing shower is to be taken.

4. Laetrile treatment: Those patients taking laetrile will have it applied 15 minutes before the scheduled treatment.

5. Herb tea: 15 minutes before the treatment a cup of hot herb tea is given.

6. Bathing suit: Upon arrival in the department the patient changes into a bathing suit.

7. Tub: From the hot shower, the patient goes to the tub. The tub is entered slowly, submerging until the shoulders are covered and a comfortable position found.

8. Tea: A second cup of herbal tea is taken upon entering the tub.

9. Cover head with towel: The head will be covered by a towel to limit heat loss.

10. Monitor temperature and pulse: Temperature and pulse will be monitored frequently as the body temperature increases.

11. Relax: The patient is encouraged to relax. As the temperature increases, breathing exercises are used, e.g.: breathe in through the nose, pulling the air in with the "stomach muscles," then out through the mouth. Swab the face, and fan with a wash cloth.

12. Time: 20-30 minutes: It takes about 20-30 minutes for the average patient to reach 103° - 104° F. On the first treatment a lower temperature is attempted (101° - 102°) to begin acclimatization. The final temperature is determined by what the patient feels he can tolerate.

13. Heat the bed: Preheat the patients bed using an electric blanket over the other blankets. Help the patient into the warmed bed and disconnect the electric blanket.

14. Stay in warm bed: The body temperature is maintained in the bed for another 15-20 minutes at which time the blankets are slowly removed, one by one. This cooling-off process will take about another 20 minutes. Upon leaving the tub and entering the bed, sips of hot herb tea are given. As the cooling-off process continues, cooler fluids (never cooler than room temperature) can be given until, at the time of completion, several glasses of orange juice are recommended.

15. Shower: When the patient returns to his room, a lukewarm shower should be used to further assist in washing off the skin. A restful afternoon is indicated. Many patients sleep for several hours following treatment. Regular meals and juices need not be interrupted.

Important Points To Be Observed With All Hydrotherapy Treatments:

- The room should be warm and free of drafts.
- Protect bedding, furniture, rugs, etc. with waterproof sheets.
- Assemble Supplies before starting procedures.
- Use care when adding hot or cold water. Avoid chilling. Patient should be dry and warm after treatment.

Clay poultice

Definition:

A soft composition, usually heated and spread on a cloth, and applied to a sore or inflamed part of the body.

Effects:

Clay powder has an adsorptive effect like that of charcoal and aids detoxification.

Indications:

Diarrhea, poison, gastrointestinal problems, inflammation, insect bites, swellings from arthritis, pain.

Procedure

1. Prepare enough warm water to mix needed amount of clay powder into a paste.
2. Apply quickly to square of clean muslin to

prevent cooling.

3. Place on area to be treated.
4. Cover with plastic and wool cloth.
5. Pin in place. Leave on overnight or until dry.
6. Remove - rub cold wet cloth over part.
7. Repeat as needed.

Chapter 2: Going Home, The Gerson Household

Follow-up medical care and laboratory monitoring

Medical consultations and the monitoring of laboratory studies are of utmost importance. Through this means, the Gerson physician can be kept up to date as he assists the patient in adjusting the various medications and the diet, and evaluating the body's response to the therapy. Continued communication with the Gerson physician also keeps the patient abreast of advances in the Gerson program.

Medical guidance is provided to the Gerson patient through your Gerson hospital's consulting office. Telephone and fax numbers will be provided through the hospital office.

Note: *Time does not usually allow correspondence in writing regarding test result information. Please use the telephone consultation program.*

Laboratory monitoring

Monitoring of blood and urine values on a continual basis is important. These laboratory tests should be repeated about every six weeks, depending upon the severity of the disease process. In the early stages with the debilitated patient, every four weeks is recommended. Before you leave the Gerson hospital your doctor will suggest a time for your next tests to be done. Copies of results should be sent to your Gerson consulting doctor.

These laboratory studies must include:

1. Complete blood count (CBC) with differential
2. Blood chemistry panel (SMAC-24 or SMA-21, etc.)
3. Analysis of urine (U/A)

These studies are monitored primarily to screen for possible infections, determine time to introduce the dairy proteins, and evaluate general organ functions such as kidney, liver and pancreas.

A single laboratory result is not definitive. A series of three results may show a trend. Routine laboratory studies have been shown not to be valid during or just after a healing reaction. The chemistry of the blood can be altered during the healing reaction. Wait at least seven to ten days after the healing reaction has cleared to have new laboratory tests done.

Outpatient follow-up checklist

✔ Approximately five weeks after you arrive home, have the following blood and urine work done:

- CBC differential
- SMAC-21 (Comprehensive Metabolic Panel Blood Chemistry Test)
- U/A (Urinalysis)

✔ Send lab rest results to your Gerson consulting physician by mail or Fax.

✔ Have your questions and concerns written down on paper next to the phone to save time. Have blank paper and a pen handy to write down your doctor's suggestions - it is not easy to remember details later.

Note: *factors for adjustment and modification of diet, medication, enemas, etc.:*

1. Length of time on therapy
2. Lab evaluation
3. Clinical information (medical)

Medication supplies

Required items for 3 month supply - Several days in advance of departure, please arrange with the hospital office for your order. Please take inventory of items before departure.

✔	Item	Qty.	Description
	Syringes	90	3cc with 22 or 23 gauge needle x 1"
	Needles	90	25 gauge x 1"
	Crude Liver	27	10cc bottles for injection
	Vit. B-12	1	30cc bottle for injection
	Thyroid	1	grain (32.4 mg), 1000 count tabs
	Lugol's	1	bottle of 1/2 strength Lugol's solution
	Penicillin	1	bottle of 100 tablets
	Potassium Compound	12	bottles, 100 grams each
	Potassium Gluconate	1	bottle
	Acidol	5	bottles of 100 caps each
	Niacin	1	bottle of 1000 tabs, 50 mg. each
	Pancreatin	1	bottle of 1000 caps, 325 mg. each
	Liver Caps	1	bottle of 1000 caps, 500 mg. each
	Ox-Bile	1	bottle
	Ion Min	1	bottle Ion Min Clay powder
	Enema Buckets	2	extra enema buckets
	Castor Oil	1	pint
	Castile Soap	1	bar of soap
	Flaxseed Oil	8	bottles
	Foley Food Mill	1	two quart size

Non-required but recommended items:

- pancreatin-extra strength, 1200 mg
- Wobe enzymes
- nelaton enema catheter
- hydrogen peroxide 30%
- organic coffee - 1 kg. bags
- charcoal tablets
- water distiller
- home ozone generator
- electric hot plate
- vaseline

Instructions for giving injections

When you return home, you will probably be administering your own injections. During your stay at The Gerson Therapy Center, injections are administered by your medical staff. Learn how to give your own injections by observing, experiencing, and asking questions.

1. Assemble items needed:

- ✔ Alcohol
- ✔ Cotton
- ✔ Syringe
- ✔ Extra Needle
- ✔ Crude liver extract
- ✔ Vitamin B-12

2. Bottle: Remove protective metal covers from rubber stopper.

3. With alcohol swab, clean tops of bottles.

4. Keep needle and syringe sterile (do not touch).

5. Turn B_{12} bottle upside down and push syringe needle through stopper. Pull out 0.1 cc (just a few drops, to the first small line on the barrel of the syringe). Withdraw needle from B_{12};. Draw 3cc of air into syringe. Turn the crude liver bottle upside down and push needle up through center of stopper. Keeping the liver extract bottle in an upside-down position, push some air into the crude liver bottle and pull some liver extract out, repeating this process until you have pulled out 3cc of liver extract (pull plunger to first line below 3cc marking to allow for B_{12}).

6. Remove and discard needle. It is now too dull for injection use.

7. Screw new needle into syringe. (Use 25 gauge 5/8" or 1" needle.) Gently tap the side of the syringe to gather bubbles to the top of the syringe. When bubbles are gathered, press plunger until a tiny bit of fluid spurts from the needle. Syringe is now ready to be used. (Put needle cover on loosely.)

8. Clean injection area well with alcohol and cotton.

Locating Injection area: Locate the ridge of your hipbone (iliac crest) where your side pants seam runs, roughly in the middle of your side. Measure down the width of two fingers and back one inch (1"). That is where the needle goes. The needle should go through the fatty tissue into the muscle. Alternate sides with each injection.

Hanson's Modification of Classic Method of Locating Upper Outer Quadrant

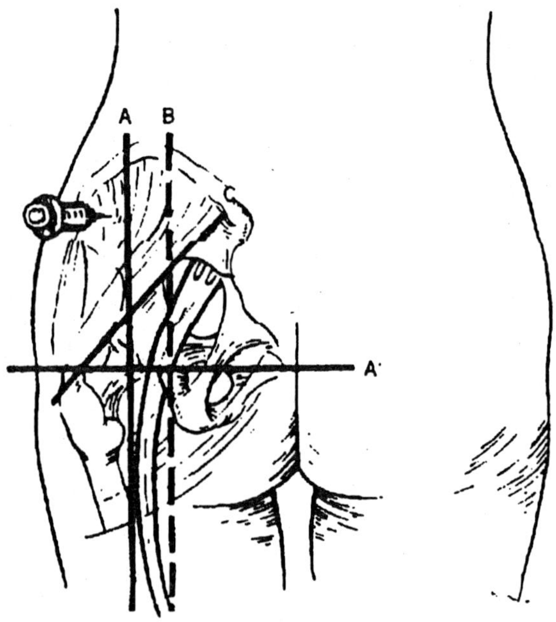

9. Spread skin and push needle in.

10. Push plunger down slowly.

11. Pull needle out and rub area with alcohol for 30 seconds. If bleeding occurs, press cotton to wound. It will stop bleeding very shortly.

12. Break needle and disassemble syringe. Keep broken needles in a small cardboard box. Tape box shut when full and discard.

13. Clean open liver and B_{12} bottles with alcohol and store in refrigerator. Protect with fresh baggie after each use. Store unopened liver extract bottles in refrigerator.

Finding organically grown food

Check the local yellow pages for health food stores and co-ops. Call and ask if they supply organically grown produce. They may know where you can go.

Contact OFPANA, Box 1078, Greenfield, MA, 10301, (413) 774-7511. Ask them for the names, addresses, and phone numbers of the organizations in your area (OCIA, CCOF, TILTH, etc.) Ask about distributors, growers, and possible retailers.

Order the *Organic Wholesaler's Directory And Yearbook* from Community Alliance with Family Farmers. It has an in-depth list of organic wholesalers by State. Once you contact the wholesalers, you can learn who their retailers are. You can contact them at Box 464, Davis, CA 95617, (916)756-8518.

Americans For Safe Food, Center for Science in the Public Interest has an organics mail order list available, should you need to order organic produce through the mail. You can contact them at 1875 Connecticut Ave NW, Suite 300, Washington, DC 20009, Tel: (202) 332-9110, Fax: (202) 265 4954,

Get certification! If produce is not clearly marked with a printed label, it is probably not organic. Demand proof.

Organic coffee information

It is just as important to use organic coffee as to use organic fruits and vegetables. If organic coffee is not used, any toxic material in the coffee such as pesticides, herbicides, fungicides, or chemical fertilizer will be readily absorbed rectally direct into the blood system. Harbor House Coffee (Organic Coffee), 12586 Foothill Blvd., Box 1879, Clearlake Oaks, CA 95423. Telephone (707) 998-4654, Toll-free: 1-888-902-6333.

Organic Certification Logos

The Gerson household: kitchen supplies

The following checklist will be found useful in arranging a household to accommodate the Gerson patient. Most items may be purchased locally at a general department store, health food store or gourmet shop.

Appliances

- ☐ Juicer (press type)
- ☐ Water distiller
- ☐ Liquid warmer: low temperature burner plate
- ☐ Second refrigerator (optional)
- ☐ Yogurt maker (optional)
- ☐ Orange juicer, reamer type
- ☐ Blender: can be used instead of rotary food mill with some recipes

Cookware

Stainless steel pots and pans with tight fitting lids

- ☐ 1 qt. saucepan
- ☐ 2 qt. saucepan
- ☐ 3 qt. saucepan
- ☐ 4 qt. saucepot
- ☐ 8 qt. saucepot
- ☐ Pyrex or Corningware baking dishes with covers

Note: *Teflon and other inert non-stick surfaces are not allowed.* ***Absolutely No Aluminum!*** *(Aluminum-clad stainless steel pots are OK).* ***No Pressure Cookers!***

Kitchen utensils

- ☐ Vegetable brushes: for scrubbing and cleaning vegetables
- ☐ Plastic cutting boards (assortment of sizes)
- ☐ Rotary food mill: for milling special soup (can use blender)
- ☐ Sixty minute timer: for juices
- ☐ Wire bristled brushes: for cleaning juicer parts
- ☐ Glass measuring cups: 1 Cup and 4 Cup
- ☐ Oven thermometer: for checking oven temperature
- ☐ Funnels: for filling jars and bottles
- ☐ Strainers: for coffee, tea
- ☐ Colander: (a perforated bowl) for straining coarse vegetables
- ☐ Mixing bowls: a set of convenient sizes
- ☐ Grater: To grate food fine to coarse
- ☐ Knives: Various sizes including 2-3 paring knives
- ☐ Measuring Spoons: for measuring small amounts
- ☐ Metal spatula
- ☐ Potato masher: Of solid wood or heavy wire for mashing foods
- ☐ Soup ladle: For serving soups
- ☐ Apple corer: to remove apple cores
- ☐ Garlic press: for crushing garlic
- ☐ Thermoses: for soup, juices, tea
- ☐ Kitchen scale: 10 or 25 lb.
- ☐ Glass storage jars: dry coffee, potassium solution, etc.
- ☐ Jar for coffee concentrate with 1 C calibration marks
- ☐ Pill container: with 6 sections

Condiments and staples

- ☐ Herbs and Spices **(see permitted spices, p. 242 in *A Cancer Therapy: Results of 50 Cases*)**
- ☐ Drip ground organic coffee
- ☐ Honey
- ☐ Organic rolled oats (old fashioned)
- ☐ Pure maple syrup
- ☐ Crude raw brown sugar (organic dried cane sugar)
- ☐ Dried fruits (soak before cooking)
- ☐ Flaxseed oil (in black bottles)
- ☐ Red wine vinegar
- ☐ Unsulphured blackstrap molasses
- ☐ Peppermint tea
- ☐ Chamomile tea
- ☐ Lemons

Paper goods

- ☐ Paper Towels
- ☐ Muslin or cheesecloth
- ☐ Toilet paper
- ☐ Juicing cloths
- ☐ Waxed paper

Bathroom supplies

- ☐ Enema Bucket
- ☐ Castile soap
- ☐ Castor oil
- ☐ Ox bile powder
- ☐ Paper towels
- ☐ Wooden spoon
- ☐ Enamel pitcher
- ☐ Toilet paper
- ☐ Toothpaste (Chloresium, Tom's, Shaklee, Waleda, unfluoridated, and without baking soda)
- ☐ Shampoo (natural shampoo, no artificial coloring or proteins added. Some brands: Nature's Gate, Tom's, Shaklee)
- ☐ Vaseline

Pollution in and around the home

Pollutants and toxins in the living environment need to be eliminated. Check your home and eliminate as many contaminants as possible:

- ☐ Asbestos
- ☐ Urea formaldehyde insulation
- ☐ Synthetic materials in rugs, draperies, bedding and clothing (use natural fibers)
- ☐ Cigarette smoke
- ☐ Pesticides and herbicides
- ☐ Fluoride in the water
- ☐ New carpeting
- ☐ Solvents, Polishes

Grocery list for a week

- ☐ Carrots, 50 lbs.
- ☐ Tomatoes, 10-15 lbs.
- ☐ Potatoes, 25 lbs.
- ☐ Onions, 20/week (purchase 25 lb. sack)
- ☐ Leeks, 2 bunches
- ☐ Beets, 5 branch tops for juice and bottoms for eating
- ☐ Green Peppers, 8 weekly
- ☐ Celery, 2-3 bunches
- ☐ Celery Root, 2 roots (if available)
- ☐ Romaine, 20 good size
- ☐ Chard, 4 bunches
- ☐ Endive, 3 heads
- ☐ Lettuce, 15 heads (red leaf, green leaf, oakleaf, butter leaf, etc.)
- ☐ Watercress, 2 bunches
- ☐ Escarole, 2-3 heads
- ☐ Parsley, 1 bunch
- ☐ Parsley root, 2 bunches (if available)
- ☐ Various vegetables, in season
- ☐ Apples 40 lbs. (pippins or granny smith apples)
- ☐ Oranges, 10-15 lbs.
- ☐ Garlic, 1 bulb
- ☐ Coffee, 3-5 Lbs.
- ☐ Distilled water, 15 gallons

***Note:** Depending on regional water supplies, various forms of water purification may be purchased or leased at considerable savings over purchased bottled water. Various combinations of distillation, carbon filtration, and reverse osmosis should be considered. Consult regional authorities.*

Water

Gerson patients need pure water, especially for coffee enemas. Most cities have bottled water businesses that deliver purified and distilled water to homes. Water can also be purified at home with reasonably priced equipment that may be purchased or rented.

Water purification equipment is everywhere now. You can get reverse osmosis units, distillers, carbon filters and more from just about anyone. People go door to door selling all sorts, sizes and combinations. Fluoride can only be removed by distillation. You should only use reverse osmosis if your tap water is not fluoridated.

Hardball sales pitch

Maybe you've seen the guy who takes a glass of your regular tap water and tests it with a "special chemical" that causes gobs of white grungy looking stuff to appear and settle to the bottom. Now he informs you that you can get all that poison out with a carbon filter, and he proves it by filtering your water and repeating the test. Voila! No grunge.

In a well researched article in their *Consumer Reports: 1992 Buying Guide Issue*, Consumers Union (CU) staff members explained that the "special chemical" is doubtless a flocculating agent that causes harmless minerals in water to precipitate. Unscrupulous sellers use this bogus water test to convince potential buyers of the unpotability of tap water in their homes.

Unsafe tap water

In fact, your tap water may be teeming with hazards, none of which would be recognized by such a "test." According to CU writers, there are more than 70,000 recognized water contaminants ranging from industrial or agricultural wastes to heavy metals and radon. Microbes are also known to flow from the household tap. If your municipal water supply is fluoridated, it is imperative that you use distilled water for all patient intake: soup, cooking, teas and coffee for enemas and drinking after castor oil.

Labs that test water

For the Gerson household, it is probably unnecessary to carry out lab tests for contaminants because of the demand for really pure water. However, friends and relatives interested in water quality issues may wish to use one of these CU listed labs:

National Testing Laboratories
6151 Wilson Mills Road
Cleveland, OH 44143
Tel.: 800-458-3330

Water Testing Laboratories
4600 Kutztown Rd.
Temple, PA 19560
Tel.: 800-433-6595

WaterTest
33 S. Commercial St.
Manchester, NH 03101
Tel.: 800-426-8378

These tests are expensive, ranging easily up to $200.

CU writers were most concerned about lead, radon, and nitrate as water contaminants. There are good reasons to remove added fluorides and chlorine, as well.

No single machine does it all

The big surprise is that no single form of water purification, tested by CU was able to remove all contaminants; not distillers; not reverse osmosis units; and not carbon filters.

In order to get really pure water, it's necessary to combine techniques. You have two choices:

1. Carbon filtration with reverse osmosis
2. Carbon filtration with distillation

Strengths and weaknesses

For practical purposes, distillers are better at organic health hazards than reverse osmosis units, but they miss the volatile ones like benzene, carbon tetrachloride and trichloroethylene. These minor differences disappear when either type of water purification is coupled with carbon filtration.

Only carbon filtration is able to remove chlorine, benzene, carbon tetrachloride, trichloroethylene, and radon. Carbon filters sound pretty good so far, but they fall apart when they get to the inorganic health hazards.

Only distillers or reverse osmosis units will take out arsenic, barium, cadmium, chromium, fluoride, lead, nitrate, and selenium.

Buy or rent?

If you are in a locale that is not serviced by a reputable water company, e.g.: Culligan, you may have to purchase equipment. Your costs may run from $500 to $1,400 for either of the effective combinations. Also, bear in mind that your costs won't end with your purchase.

Distillers typically draw 1500 Watts, and electricity is expensive. Extrapolating CU writers' numbers, it looks like five gallons of water will cost $1.50 on the utility bill. For patients, the electricity cost alone may run approximately $30 per month.

Carbon filters are replaced frequently, on the order of every six months for high volume usage. Replacement costs run from $5 to $100.

Reverse osmosis units allow up to 80% of water to flow by the membrane and down the drain. When it's time to replace the membrane, usually once a year, costs range from $45 to $234.

If, after reading the above, you still want to own your own gear, we recommend that you use the CU ratings guide to make good choices within a reasonable budget.

You may choose to rent

On the other hand, you may choose to rent. Many companies rent and maintain an under-the-sink combination reverse osmosis and carbon filtration unit. The customer pays no replacement costs for filters or membranes. A test light signals when the unit needs servicing. Most units make plenty of water, allowing up to five gallons per day when needed.

Finding a vendor

Water companies can be found in the Yellow Pages and most offer a filtration service.

The quality of tap water almost everywhere, is less than acceptable for the Gerson Therapy. Fortunately, purification units are available, affordable, and effective.

Schedule for the day

The following is an example of one way to arrange your schedule to do the Gerson Therapy at home. This schedule was set up for a regular day on full therapy including 13 juices and 5 coffee enemas. Whoever is doing the kitchen work should allow about 10-15 minutes to prepare a juice and to clean up the juicer, so start making the juices about 15 minutes before the hour. Juices are followed in this list by the medications (in parentheses) which may be added. Please do not exceed daily total medication levels prescribed by your physicians.

Getting organized

If at all possible, have someone at home organize things before you leave the Gerson hospital. They will need to:

1. Locate and purchase organic produce.
2. Locate and purchase organic coffee.
3. Set up the Juicer.
4. Reorganize the kitchen (see list) paying special attention to remove all sprays, poisons, perfumed items, and aluminum pots and pans.
5. Clear the counters. Get everything off but the juicer and the cutting boards.
6. Knives: You will be doing a lot of cutting so make sure the knives are sharp.
7. Purified Water: See previous page 15 for information on obtaining purified water.
8. You may need to rearrange the bedroom and bathroom to accommodate coffee enemas. A bench will be necessary if movement is impaired.

Daily Schedule - Example

AM	**Morning**
7:00	Rise and shine
7:15	Coffee Break (Be sure to eat a bite of fruit before enema)
7:45	1) Start oatmeal and coffee concentrate 2) Make citrus juice (Lugol's and potassium) 3) Sort medications for the day
8:00	Eat breakfast (Orange juice + meds)
8:30	1) Wash the vegetables and fruits that you will use for the day's juices and meals 2) Strain the coffee 3) Start the Special (Hippocrates) soup (see recipe, pg. 80)
9:00	Green juice (potassium)
9:30	Carrot-Apple juice (Lugol's and potassium)
10:00	Carrot-Apple juice (Lugol's and potassium)
11:00	Carrot juice (2 Liver tablets) Prepare potatoes and vegetables for lunch
11:15	Coffee Break
PM	**Afternoon/Evening**
12:00	1) Green juice (potassium) 2) Prepare lunch Salad Start vegetables and watch that they do not burn
1:00	Special (Hippocrates) soup (see recipe, pg. 80) Eat lunch Carrot-Apple juice (Lugol's and potassium)
2:00	Green juice (potassium)
3:00	Carrot juice (w/2 Liver tablets)
4:00	Coffee Break + Carrot juice (w/Liver tablets)
5:00	Carrot-Apple juice (2 Liver tablets)
6:00	Green juice (potassium) Prepare dinner, salad, potatoes, vegetables, carrot apple juice, etc.
7:00	Eat dinner + Carrot-Apple juice + Meds
8:00	Coffee Break Put together a fruit plate to nibble on through the night
10:00	Coffee Break (Be sure to eat some fruit first)
AM	**Late Night/Early Morning**
3:00	Coffee Break, if ordered by physician. (Eat first)

Chapter 3: General Procedures, Common Reactions and Personal Care

Enema Recipes

It is very important for all fluids that are placed in the rectum to be sterile. Use boiled water only! Be sure you allow fluids to cool to body temperature before placing in rectum. **(For further information, see pp. 247-248, *A Cancer Therapy: Results of Fifty Cases*)**

Recipe: Coffee Enema, Recommended

This recipe is used full strength: do not dilute!

- 3 Rounded Tbsp. coffee grounds (not instant)
- 1 Quart distilled water

Boil 3 minutes uncovered to drive off oils; then cover, lower heat and simmer an additional 15 minutes. Strain and allow to cool. Add distilled water to make a full quart. Use at body temperature.

Recipe: Coffee Enema, Concentrate

Place in saucepan

- 1 Cup coffee grounds (not instant)
- 1 Quart distilled water

Boil 3 minutes uncovered. Cover, lower heat and simmer for 15 minutes. Strain into 1 quart jar, allowing grounds to drain well. Add distilled water to make a full quart. **For convenience:** Mark the jar indicating 1 Cup increments. **Diluting:** This recipe makes enough concentrate for 4 enemas (1 cup concentrate plus 3 Cups boiled/distilled water) **Storage:** This concentrate will keep in a refrigerator for up to 2 days.

Note: *The physicians recommend that coffee concentrate be used only as an alternative to the above recipe for convenience when traveling.*

Apply enema following instructions on page 191 of *A Cancer Therapy: Results of Fifty Cases*, or see page 19 in this handbook.

Chamomile Tea Enema:

Use full strength and according to your doctor's advice. Retain the tea enema for about five minutes. After release, immediately start the coffee enema. In severe problems, chamomile concentrate can be added to all coffee enemas.

Recipe: Chamomile Enema, Single

- 4 Tbsp. Chamomile flowers, dried
- 1 Quart distilled water

Boil 5 minutes, and strain.
Use when cooled to body temperature.

Recipe: Chamomile Concentrate

- 1 Cup Chamomile flowers, dried
- 2 Cups distilled water

Simmer 10 minutes in covered saucepan. Strain and press chamomile flowers to extrude fluid. If some has boiled away, add distilled water to make 1 pint. **Storage:** Keep in covered glass bottle no longer than 3 days. **To Use:** Pour 4 oz. concentrate into enema bucket and fill with distilled water. **Recipe makes enough concentrate for 4 enemas.**

NOTE: *Some confusion has existed because of an apparent contradiction between chamomile enema instructions on page 194 and page 248 of Gerson's A Cancer Therapy: Results of Fifty Cases. Actually, the recipes are consistent. Page 194 includes instructions for use of a chamomile concentrate as well as directions for preparation of a single dose. Page 248 contains instructions for both preparation and use of chamomile concentrate . In both cases, the ratio of chamomile flowers (in tablespoons) to total ounces of water will be the same: 4 Tbsp. / 32 oz. enema.*

Please understand that the concentrate is prepared by using 1 Tbsp. of chamomile flowers for each ounce of water: one cup (16 Tbsp.) chamomile flowers boiled in 1 pint (16 oz) water makes four doses. Gerson's "glass" equals 8 oz, just as with your juices. One half glass equals 4 oz.

Enema Procedure

Definition:

An enema by definition, is the introduction of solutions into the rectum and colon in order to stimulate bowel activity and to cause emptying of the lower intestine.

Coffee enemas should be administered by having the patient lie on the right side.

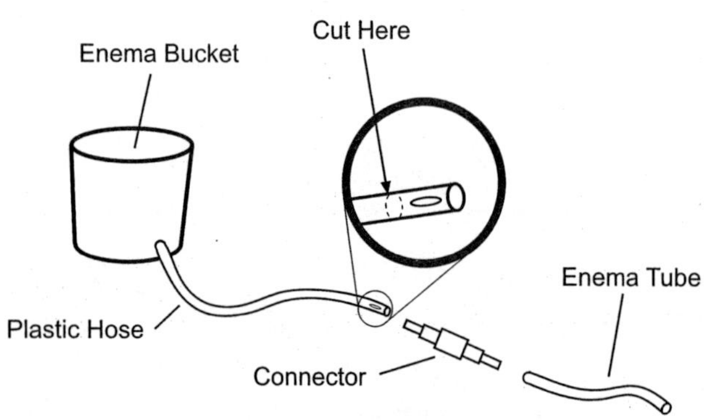

To connect bucket, tube and connector:
The enema bucket comes with a clear plastic hose which has a hole at the front and one on the side. You cut off the tip to eliminate the side opening.

You order a small plastic connector plus a soft rubber tube (catheter) both available from STAT. S.A. Put one end of the connector onto the cut end of the plastic enema tube: the other end into the wide opening of the rubber catheter.

Some patients find it difficult to retain 32 oz. of the liquid, you may want to start with 24 oz. and later, slowly increase the amount of fluid.

Before you start your coffee enema, eat a small piece of fruit to activate the gastric tract If enema is taken on an empty stomach, some people may experience problems.

Note: *More information on enemas is available in* A Cancer Therapy: Results of Fifty Cases *on pages 191 and 247 and in* Gerson Healing Newsletter *Vol. 10, No. 4, pg. 6, and Gerson Healing Newsletter #13, pg. 1.*

Enema Reactions and Remedies

Intestinal Spasms and Cramping:

These frequently painful symptoms are caused by strong irritation to the intestinal tract and lead to problems with the enemas. It becomes difficult to instill the full 32 oz. of coffee solution, difficult to hold the enema the full 12-15 minutes or, on the other hand, the enema becomes trapped and cannot be released. Following is a list of possible remedies which have proved useful to patients:

Check The Enema Technique:

Be sure that the tip of the enema tube is inserted five to eight inches past the anal sphincter. Do not try to force the tube into the colon. The temperature of the enema solution must be body temperature. Don't raise the enema bucket too high. If the flow is too rapid it can set up spasms. About eighteen to twenty-four inches is the correct bucket height. Even at that height, spasms can occur. If so, immediately lower the bucket to allow the flow to back up a few inches into the tube to relieve the pressure. After 20 to 30 seconds slowly start raising the bucket toward the original level. The flow can also be controlled by pinching the tube with your fingers or adjusting the plastic ring to a partially closed position. It may take some time to get the enema completely instilled, but this is acceptable.

Heat Over The Abdomen:

This can be applied by a heating pad. Mild heat has a calming effect on the irritated, hyperactive intestinal tract.

Add Potassium Compound To The Enema:

Potassium compound solution helps relieve spasms by supplying potassium to the depleted intestinal tract. It can also help to promote bile flow when given rectally. This solution is the same as that used in the juices. The dosage is two Tbsp. in each enema. Procedure should be discontinued after 10 days to 2 weeks.

Lower The Dosage:

This can be accomplished by either using less coffee concentrate in each enema, or by using only part of a prepared enema. Please consult with physician.

Back To Back Enemas:

When the first enema is "clutched" and the abdomen congested, a second enema may be taken "back to back" with the first. Potassium compound solution (see above) may be added to the second enema to promote effectiveness. Another potentially valuable aid is hydrogen peroxide (1-2 tsp. of 3%) added to the second enema. Chamomile concentrate may be added to counter the irritating effects of either peroxide or potassium taken by rectum.

CAUTION: If you run into chronic problems, please do not resort to a long series of consecutive enemas (use no more than 2 back to back). At least four hours must be allowed between back to back enemas in most cases. Please be in touch with your physician.

Castor Oil Enema: *may also be used in some cases if a back to back enema is "clutched." Castor oil enemas are extremely pushy and should be used cautiously - generally only one in a 24 hour period. Consult your physician.*

Colds and Flus

There is quite a serious problem presently in the general population, consisting of depressed immune systems. We are seeing a constant increase in infections that were virtually unknown two decades ago: AIDS, 'chronic fatigue syndrome' (CFS, or Epstein-Barr), genital herpes, hepatitis of all kinds and Candida (yeast infections). Other infectious diseases that once seemed to have almost disappeared, such as tuberculosis, and even syphilis, are making a threatening comeback.

It must be assumed that our poor general nutrition, together with excess consumption of fats, proteins and salt, has caused this health problem. Obviously, patients suffering from cancer have a seriously weakened immune system - since a fully functioning immune response is capable of protecting the body from ever developing cancer. So, we know that in all cancer patients, we have a problem if they 'catch' cold or develop a flu. Even after a few months on the Gerson Therapy, which among other things restores the immune system, the former cancer patient does not yet have a good defense against cold and flu viruses. For that reason, much care has to be taken to protect the recovering patient from visitors, children or other household members who have colds. They should be completely segregated from the patient. Friends or visitors with colds should be urgently requested not to visit, or, if they have come into the house, the patient should quietly, even unsociably disappear behind his/her bedroom door.

If a recovering patient does develop a cold or flu, at the very first signs, he should take penicillin (other antibiotics if he is allergic to penicillin) together with the 'triad' (one Aspirin, one 50 mg. Niacin, one 500 mg. Vitamin C), at least once every six hours for as long as symptoms are present, plus one day. It is also wise to gargle with chamomile tea in which you use 1/2 ounce of a 3% solution of hydrogen peroxide, at least three times a day. A very warm bath with at least 4 pints of 3% hydrogen peroxide twice a day is extremely helpful. Be sure that the patient is not chilled upon leaving the bath and immediately goes into a warm bed. A cold should be treated with great respect since it can cause recurrence of tumors. If you report to your Gerson consulting doctor with possible regrowth of tumors, be sure you mention whether or not you had a cold or flu in the recent past, and whether you have overcome it.

Because of the seriousness of possible colds, it is suggested on the list of medications to take home, that you take penicillin with you. If, at the very first symptoms of a cold, you first have to go to a doctor for a prescription, or ask for penicillin to be mailed to you - it will be much too late to take it. It is mainly used to avoid opportunistic germs from aggravating the virus infection - but you need to have it on hand in case of need. Do not use it for any other reason.

Exercise

Dr. Gerson felt very strongly that a cancer patient just starting on the therapy, urgently needs rest. He even had patients who were not particularly debilitated, stay in bed for a full six weeks! The Gerson Therapy itself speeds up the metabolism, and that requires energy. This extra energy requirement often causes patients starting the treatment to be tired. This is an urgent message from the body to rest! Do not force exercise when you are tired. It will not 'build you up' at all; on the contrary, it will slow down or stop the healing process if you waste your energy.

Early on in the treatment, it is a good practice to do some trampolining. A little 'rebounder' is quite inexpensive, and can be very helpful. In the beginning, use it only by lifting your heel and bending your knees - don't jump. Also, it is best to use it for only 30 seconds at a time, but several times a day - as often as 5-6 times. This very mild exercise stimulates lymphatic circulation and also helps to overcome pain, especially bone pain. But, again, don't overdo or exhaust yourself.

When patients first return home, they usually feel much better, but not yet strong. It is extremely important that they do not immediately jump into their jobs or housework - since the Therapy with all the foods and juices is very labor intensive. The patient needs continued rest and HELP. Usually, after about three months, energy returns. That, too, can be a period of danger: when the patient is recovering and feels energy again, he/she may well begin strenuous activities - overexerting himself, and stopping the healing. Do not overdo. As your energy returns, you can begin some very mild exercise: a five minute walk (not in extreme heat or cold). This can soon be extended to 8-10 minutes, but, if the patient is very tired, stop, and go back to the last amount of walking that didn't exhaust you. Increase the time for a walk very slowly if you can easily handle it. More strenuous exercise (tennis, squash) must be avoided for a year or so. Try to avoid walking on or near a golf course, as the grass is heavily sprayed with toxic chemicals. Swimming is a problem: all chlorinated pools must be completely avoided and ocean water is too salty for the patient. So what remains? A clean mountain stream or lake. "Clean" means that there are no factories that drain chemicals into the water above the place where you swim. And, of course, the weather must be mild or warm, so the patient is not chilled. One of our recovered breast cancer patients in Carmel, California, after two years on the therapy and total recovery, won several tennis tournaments. Just be patient and heal first!

Flare-ups and reactions

Notes from a lecture by Dr. Dan Rogers, M.D.

Definition of Flare-up/Reaction: A response by the body in general, and the immune system in particular, causing an increase in detoxification and healing processes.

Causes: The causes can be many; the body's attempt to rid itself of dead and diseased tissue and cells, eliminate toxins of all types, and rebuild healthy cells and tissues.

Flare-ups may include any of the following symptoms:

Flu-like symptoms:

General aches and pains, sore muscles and joints, or an "achy all over feeling" are fairly common in most patients. The duration of these symptoms is usually 24-48 hours. Usually self-limited, but may require mild definitive treatment.

Rx: Treat symptomatically including clay/castor oil packs, pain triad, hydrotherapy, and/or bed rest.

Nausea:

This reaction may be intense, lasting for several days. Usually self-limited.

Rx: Treat symptomatically. Increase intake of peppermint tea and oatmeal. May need to decrease oral solid intake or exchange it for raw grated apples, applesauce, raw grated carrots, mashed banana, watermelon, etc. Also, change juice composition by adding up to 50% gruel per juice. May also give gruel straight.

Vomiting:

Does not occur in most cases. If it does occur it usually lasts 24 hours or less. Some cases can be intense and of longer duration, requiring definitive treatment, especially when complicated by other body fluid loss (such as diarrhea), or in a patient with reduced body mass (i.e. child, cachexia, etc.).

Rx: Increase peppermint tea intake to as much as 1 gallon or more and substitute oatmeal for regular meals when needed. May need to decrease oral solid intake or exchange it for raw grated apples, applesauce, raw grated carrots, mashed banana, watermelon, etc. Also change juice composition by adding up to 50% gruel per juice. May also give gruel straight. Juices not taken orally can be given rectally as a retention enema. If emesis lasts longer than 24 hours, or if severe, definitive treatment may be required including antiemetics (oral, I.M., or I.V.), and I.V. fluids. Serum electrolyte and acid/base levels need to be carefully monitored. If vomiting bile (green, bitter) reduce coffee enemas to 1 or 2 a day and take chamomile enemas between coffee enemas.

Diarrhea:

Frequent passage of unformed, watery bowel movements. If it occurs it is usually self-limiting, lasting 24-48 hours. If it persists any longer, definitive treatment may be required, especially when complicated by other body fluid loss such as vomiting, or in a patient with reduced body mass (i.e.: child, cachexia, etc.)

Rx: Treat symptomatically. As an initial measure, combine 1/8 tsp. potassium gluconate and 1/4 tsp. clay in peppermint tea, to be taken every 2-4 hours. If particularly severe or lasting longer than 24-48 hours, antispasmotics (i.e.: polvo mixto, lomotil, etc.) may be needed. Also, routinely do lab testing, e.g. ova and parasites, stool culture and sensitivity, serum electrolytes, etc. I.V. fluids may be necessary, especially if diarrhea is complicated by increased loss of other body fluids.

Pain:

May be prodromal (i.e.: signaling a flare-up) starting as much as 48-72 hours prior to reaction. Usually self-limiting. Duration up to 72 hours post reaction. May require definitive Rx.

Rx: Treat symptomatically. Use increased enemas, clay/castor oil packs and pain triad as first treatment of choice. Laetrile (Amigdalin) is a good Rx alternative especially with bony metastases. Hydrotherapy works well with many types of pain. Acupuncture, Neural therapy with lidocaine also works well. May need triad (1 Aspirin, 1 Niacin 50 mg., 1 Vitamin C 500 mg.), etc., depending upon the type of pain and location.

Chills and Fever:

May last 24-48 hours, usually self-limited. For the most part should be treated with physical means. Areas of precaution include high fevers (greater than 104° F.) for a period greater than 2 hours, and patients with reduced body mass (i.e.: child, cachexia, etc.).

Rx: For chills, use physical means as first treatment of choice. Put the patient to bed, warm patient with blankets, pajamas, etc. May also enjoy warm bath, hot herb tea, etc. Bed rest is required.

For fever, also use physical means as first treatment of choice. Reduce amount of constrictive clothing, remove most blankets, but maintain normal environmental temperatures. Use vinegar/alcohol rub down, cool water rub down, damp cloth on neck/forehead, etc. Bed rest is necessary. If the patient's temperature continues to rise, cool chamomile tea/coffee/water enemas may be needed. Also, cool baths with up to full body immersion may be used. If fever is still rising, the pain triad, with emphasis on aspirin, may be employed. Try to avoid the use of any stronger antipyretic agents, except for very unusual circumstances. Careful monitoring of the patient is ESSENTIAL if physical means are to be successful in controlling fever, especially if body temperature remains at 104° F or more. If physical means plus aspirin and careful monitoring do not control fever at a manageable level, definitive treatment must be employed.

Foul smells:

This general category includes breath, body odor, smelly enemas, etc. At least one of these symptoms is fairly common in patients during their first reactions. They are self-limiting, lasting the duration of the reaction, and up to 48 hours post reaction. No special precautions need to be taken, except for the comfort of the patient and any visitors.

Rx: ***Breath:*** brush teeth several times per day. Eat garlic. Drink extra juice/tea. ***Body Odor:*** bathe and change clothes often. Vinegar/alcohol rubdown. Drink extra juice/tea. ***Enema odor:*** increase number of enemas, including castor oil (check with your physician). Instruct everyone to leave the room at enema time and open the bathroom windows, even in the winter. May need to repaint the room.

Depression:

This symptom is very common to many patients, especially during the first several reactions. It is due in part to the toxins released into the blood, reacting in the brain and effecting its functions. It may be a prodromal sign of an upcoming reaction, occurring as much as 72 hours before the reaction starts. It worsens as the reaction occurs, and may last up to 72 hours following the flare-up. It is usually self-limiting. The patient especially needs as much extra TLC (tender loving care) as possible at this time.

Rx: Treat symptomatically. Lots of support, TLC, encouragement, companion and family support are especially critical here.

Jaundice:

Duration usually limited to 48 hours, post flare-up.

Rx: No definitive treatment. Increase juices and enemas.

Note: *Remember flare-ups can consist of one or more of the above symptoms, and perhaps all of them.*

Laboratory Test Changes

Almost any lab value is susceptible to change during flare-ups. Especially sensitive to change are serum values such as electrolytes, Alkaline Phosphatase, GGT, GGP, SGOT, etc. A complete blood count and differential may show a relatively higher number of leukocytes and an increase in the lymphocyte count if it was low before the flare-up began, or a decrease in the lymphocyte count if it was high before the reaction started. Also, urinalysis shows trace amounts of albumin and a greater amount of sodium excretion. If your blood/urinalysis tests were done within 3 days of a reaction, be sure to tell your doctor. Your doctor may otherwise misinterpret the results.

Cosmetics and Sunscreen

Cosmetics

All substances which go on the skin, at best clog pores, keeping the skin from breathing and eliminating toxins. At worst, these materials are absorbed into the blood stream and damage the patient. While on the intensive therapy, the patient should refrain from using any skin lotions, creams, and ointments whatsoever. Especially, women need to refrain from using lipstick which is regularly licked off the lips and therefore ingested. Sometimes, women complain that their lips are dry or raw if they do not use lipstick. This is often due to the lipstick. If the patient refrains from its use for a few days, and instead uses a little Vaseline, the lips 'heal' and will feel normal.

We feel very strongly about any underarm anti-perspirant or deodorant. All these are harmful, even if purchased in a 'health food store.' Many contain aluminum, and other chemicals which should never go to block lymph passages underarm. They not only block but are absorbed and toxic. The passages should be clear and open for elimination of toxic perspiration. If sweat is smelly, wash frequently and keep the lymph passages open. To block them is to force the toxic materials back into the lymph passages, causing new harm. Once the body is well detoxified, it will not have any unpleasant smell.

Nail polish keeps the nails from breathing. Do not use it while on the Gerson Therapy; nor any artificial nails. If you are wearing it at the hospital, a nurse will provide you with nail polish remover.

We need not mention permanents or hair dyes, since these are mentioned on the list of forbidden items in ***A Cancer Therapy: Results of Fifty Cases*, p. 238**. However, hair sprays, lacquers with acetone solvents, are also very harmful and have to be avoided. On the therapy, your hair will become healthier and have natural 'body'. You will not need some of the toxic cosmetics.

Sunscreen

Dr. Gerson did not want patients to be exposed to sun, nor to sunbathe. During the last few years, it has become fashionable to recommend 'sunscreen' because many doctors claim sunlight can cause skin cancer. Dr. Gerson's reason for recommending patients avoid sunlight is that it is radiation, it is wearying and irritating; so the patient must avoid it. Sunscreen is not the answer. On the contrary: the latest information has it, the sunscreen which people are supposed to use and put on their children's skin becomes a carcinogen (cancer causing agent) when exposed to the sun! If you are going out, wear a long-sleeved shirt, preferably white cotton, or a blouse. Use a hat with a wide brim or visor to protect your face. You need not stay indoors altogether when the weather is sunny. Just don't expose yourself without clothes, to 'sunbathe'. It is always suggested that you take in fresh air, in the shade, under a tree or umbrella. If you are using the sun 'to warm you', rather use extra covers, sweaters, coats or blankets, but stay in the shade.

Dental Hygiene and Care

Toothpaste

***Extremely Important:* Never use toothpaste with fluoride or baking soda!**

Dental Abscesses

A very important consideration for success on the Gerson Therapy is the need to clear any possible dental root abscess. Sometimes, these abscesses cause no symptoms and the patient is not aware of them. Also some patients are overly concerned about X-rays, to the point that they even refuse the small amount of radiation used to diagnose possible dental problems. That is a mistake. The amount of radiation is not harmful; but the possible existence of dental root canal infections or abscesses will negate the effectiveness of the Gerson Therapy. Sometimes seriously damaged or infected teeth have to be removed in order to eliminate the constant re-infection caused by these toxins in the mouth. Please check your teeth and make sure that there are no dental problems as you start on the Therapy.

Silver-Mercury Amalgam Fillings

Many of our patients and readers are informed about the dangers of silver-amalgam fillings. These consist of a mixture of metals that can contain up to 50% mercury. The problem, of course, is that mercury is a highly toxic heavy metal, with a powerful effect on the central nervous system. Over the course of 20 years, it has been shown that up to 95% of the mercury can leach out of the fillings into the system and into circulation. Some people are a great deal more sensitive to this circulating mercury than others. It has been shown to cause Multiple Sclerosis in some patients. When the silver amalgam fillings were removed, the patients recovered. Other people have had silver fillings in their teeth for many years with no apparent problems.

Baking Soda

Your dentist can cause you considerable trouble if he recommends that you brush your teeth with baking soda. The chemical name for baking soda is sodium bicarbonate. Sodium is readily absorbed through the mucus membranes in the mouth and quickly enters the blood stream. A patient who came to us with colon cancer was completely cleared of cancer after about ten months on the therapy. She continued the therapy faithfully, as she had been instructed. Nevertheless, after another six months or so, she had a new malignant lesion in her colon. When she returned to the Gerson Therapy hospital, upon intensive questioning, it turned out her dentist had suggested she brush her teeth with baking soda. She did – and her tumor returned. When she stopped this practice, she healed again!

We need to warn our patients not to follow such dentists' instructions. Also, please note that **A Cancer Therapy: Results of Fifty Cases, on p. 238**, states on the list of forbidden items not to use baking soda also for gargling, etc. The above patient did not remember or check on this before following her dentist's instructions. Please also note that many brands of toothpaste presently contain baking soda - since dentists recommend it. Please do not use such toothpastes.

Root Canals

An entirely different situation exists when patients have been treated by their dentist with "root canal" fillings. In order to treat the root, the dentist has to drill any loose or infected material from the canal which houses the nerve. But when the nerve is dead and removed, the tooth also dies. A wonderful book called *The Root Canal Cover-Up*, published by Dr. George E. Meinig, DDS, F.A.C.D. in 1993 gives the extensive and detailed research done by Dr. Weston A. Price, DDS, F.A.C.D., early this century. Dr. Meinig for many years headed the group of dentists engaged in doing root canals. He also states he did many hundreds himself. However, when he became aware of the dangers inherent in this treatment, he incorporated his new findings in his practice and now spends his time and energies in making the public, as well as dentists, aware of the research.

The first indication of problems due to root canals came from a patient who was bedfast and virtually paralyzed due to rheumatoid arthritis, for some reason, her root canal filled tooth was removed, although it looked healthy, and after some months, she could walk and her health was totally restored. But Dr. Price took the extracted tooth, sterilized it thoroughly, and implanted it under the skin of a rabbit. Within 5 days, the rabbit was suffering with severe rheumatoid arthritis, and in 10 days it died of the disease.

Subsequently, many other patients had root canal filled teeth extracted: some suffering from kidney disease, others from heart disease, and many more with arthritis. In virtually all cases, the patients showed considerable improvement, to even total recovery, after the offending teeth were removed. But, again, many more times. Dr. Price implanted the teeth under the skin of rabbits. In each case. the tooth removed from the patient caused the patient's disease in the rabbit. Dr. Price went even further to try to clear the apparently infectious material from the extracted teeth: he autoclaved them (sterilized by steam pressure, usually at 250 degrees F or 121°C). This made no difference: the rabbits with the sterilized tooth implanted still developed the disease and died, usually within 10 days. Then Dr. Price implanted a healthy tooth under the skin of a rabbit. The rabbit lived without showing any signs of problems for about 15 years, its normal life span.

The underlying problem is very interesting: when the nerve is removed from a tooth, it is no longer living, nor is it supplied with nutrients. It is dead. However, the normal structure of the tooth includes tiny 'canules' (similar to capillaries in every human tissue) that carry nutrients to the living tooth. Once the tooth is dead, nutrients stop circulating through these canules, instead they become infested with germs and viruses. Not only that, but the filling of the nerve canal shrinks a tiny little bit, enough for more bacteria and viruses to lodge there, too. None of this shows on X-rays. A dead tooth is thus a potent source of bacterial and viral toxins and infections that can spread throughout the system. Many people with a good immune system and powerful defenses, can live with this constant source of trouble without showing any symptoms. Careful X-rays in many cases show that with time "cavitation" (hollowing out of the surrounding jaw bone) occurs around the root canal treated tooth. As the resistant patient ages or is weakened by accidents, colds and flu, or severe stress, the ability to overcome this 'focal infection' is reduced and can either cause or contribute to cause severe chronic disease.

In view of the above, it will not come as a surprise that we urgently suggest patients remove any tooth (or teeth) with root canal fillings.

A German physician. Dr. Josef Issels, heard a lecture by Dr. Gerson back in the 1950's and subsequently successfully used alternative treatments in helping many cancer patients. Dr. Issels spent some time at the Gerson Therapy Center and also pointed out the severe damage caused by root canal fillings. He further stated that he refused to treat any cancer patient who did not allow all 'devitalized' (dead) teeth to be removed. He explained that he could not obtain good results without this procedure.

As this is something that is appearing more and more often in our patients, we recommend that this be discussed with your physician if you have had root canal work done in the past.

Some dentists are now claiming that newly available materials they use in the root canal are "safe." Do not allow any root canals to be performed, as it is not the dental material, but the dead tooth that causes the problem.

Dental Anesthesia for the Gerson Patient

There are several things to remember when it comes to dental anesthesias. On the one hand, the Gerson patient since s/he is well detoxified, has a higher threshold of pain - so average pain 'doesn't hurt as much'. On the other hand, a Gerson patient is also much more sensitive to drugs and, under certain circumstances, the full average dose (2cc) of Xylocaine (or other pain killer drug) could cause serious problems. It is important that the patient advise his dentist as follows:

1. Compound the anesthesia drug without epinephrine
2. Use no more than 1/3 of the average dose
3. Start to work promptly. If a 20 minute wait is allowed for the drug to 'take' it will have worn off.

Milk Proteins

After a period of about 6 weeks on the full intensive therapy, Dr. Gerson allowed cancer patients to add modified milk proteins to their diet. Your Gerson doctor may suggest a different amount of time before allowing the addition of milk products.

It is important that milk products be:

1. Fat free (not low fat)
2. Soured (pre-digested, such as in yogurt or 'pot cheese')
3. Salt-free

In his book, *A Cancer Therapy: Results of Fifty Cases*, Dr. Gerson describes these milk proteins as 'buttermilk and pot cheese'. Unfortunately, at the present time, these products are not readily available as originally prescribed. Consequently, the currently available products cannot be used by patients on the Gerson Therapy. The buttermilk which Dr. Gerson prescribed was true, churned buttermilk. This was totally fat-free through the churning process, and contained no additives. This type of buttermilk is no longer available anywhere, as far as we know. On the other hand, present day buttermilk is 'cultured' and is usually made from left-over milk, treated with thickeners, flavoring agents, and even salt, as shown in the list of ingredients. This is not usable for a Gerson patient and could cause harm. Unless you have your own churn, or are close to a milk farmer who churns butter and has buttermilk left from his processing, you cannot use ("cultured") buttermilk while on the Gerson Therapy.

The problem of 'pot cheese' is even more complex. Dr. Gerson's patients, some 40-50 years ago, had access to a non-fat, unsalted large curd type of cottage cheese. This, too, is no longer available. Cottage cheese, on the other hand, is salted and 'creamed' (cream added). You may see some which is labeled "low fat", but this contains a minimum of 2% butterfat (too much) and is quite heavily salted. The "regular" cottage cheese contains 4% butterfat plus salt. Neither is acceptable for the Gerson patient.

The only way that patients can use 'cottage cheese' is if they are able to obtain skim milk and allow it to curdle (see Appendix III: Recipes, pg. 98) and pass it through several layers of cheese cloth, or preferably through some porous tea towel, to separate the curds from the whey.

We saw one lady who had originally shown exceptionally dramatic results with the Gerson Therapy, eating 'cottage cheese' at home. This was a hard cheese, possibly made as part of a 'cottage industry', and sold as cottage cheese. Hard cheeses are especially harmful: they usually contain up to 40% (!) butterfat, and are heavily salted. Naturally, this lady, too, experienced regrowth of tumors, until she stopped using this cheese.

We had another patient who had done very well on the Gerson Therapy and most of his tumors were gone or were reduced. When his doctor allowed him to have yogurt, he could only find "low fat" yogurt, and he decided that was okay for him. In a short time, his tumors were growing again and he came back to the Gerson Therapy Hospital to find out what the problem was. In only a few days on the full intensive therapy in Mexico, his tumors were again much smaller. Then he received the results of an analysis he had ordered of his low-fat yogurt. The result showed a fat content of this low fat' yogurt of 3.2% butterfat - enough to start tumors growing!

Other problems occur with yogurt. It has to be non-fat and unflavored. Some patients are trying their best to do right, and look for raw, unpasteurized milk yogurt. Be careful. You will possibly find raw goat's milk yogurt, and think you have it made. Not so. Goat's milk is, by nature, homogenized, and it is difficult to remove the cream – so, it is full of fat. We lost one patient because the care-giver was not aware of the danger of raw goat's milk yogurt.

Please be careful, don't go by names, but by ingredients. Cottage cheese or yogurt should contain no added salt and no fat. Some patients have expressed doubt about their yogurt when its "contents" label showed that it contained a small amount of sodium. Please understand that all milk (and vegetables, too, by the way) naturally contain a little sodium. So, if you see sodium listed under 'contents', don't worry. It should not show under 'ingredients' since this would mean that salt was added.

Occasionally, you may be able to find 'Farmer's Cheese', which contains no fat and no salt and would be acceptable. (Check your labels!) Also, some dairies produce "Baker's Cheese" to be used in baking pastries such as Cheese Danish. If this baker's cheese contains no salt or fat it may be used, whipped up with some non-fat yogurt and onions, garlic or chives - since it is quite lacking in flavor without additions. Also, Safeway used to produce cheese for the same purpose, called "Dry Curd." This is also free of salt and fat and can be mixed with onions, garlic, etc. and can be a delicious spread for baked potatoes and vegetables; or with a little maple syrup or honey, it can be used over stewed fruit, or as a sauce with some dessert.

Very rarely, a patient is lactose intolerant and cannot handle any milk products. Your doctor may advise you to take spirulina, blue-green manna, or bee pollen. This can also sometimes cause allergic reactions. If you are trying it, use just a few grains at first, and add a few at a time before reaching your prescribed amount. If it causes you any allergic reaction, don't use it.

Chapter 4: Psychological Considerations for the Gerson Patient

by Beata Bishop

According to a brief but precise definition, in holistic medicine the physician treats the patient, not the disease. This certainly applies to the Gerson Therapy which heals by restoring the health of the whole body, rather than concentrate an a specific complaint. But its powerful effects extend to the patient's non-physical self as well. In order to make the Gerson program fully holistic, the psychological aspects of healing must also be considered.

Body and mind are two sides of one coin. They sicken together and must be healed together. Whatever affects the one will affect the other. Our task is to evoke the patient's self-healing potential and make sure that some disregarded psychological problem does not sabotage the therapeutic process.

There is now solid scientific evidence to prove that our moods, emotions and general outlook have a direct and measurable impact on our immune system. The proof comes from psycho-neuro-immunology (PNI), a new medical specialty which has been rapidly developing since the late seventies, thanks to a better understanding of brain chemistry and of the subtle connections that exist on the cellular level within the body. In a nutshell, the limbic system of the brain and the central nervous system release certain hormones that fit into receptor sites all over the body, causing them to release various secretions. The quality of the hormones and the secretion determines whether the immune system is boosted or weakened, switched on or off; and that quality, in turn, depends on our emotions, beliefs and prevailing psychological orientation.

A positive, hopeful, determined attitude strengthens immune competence, while despair negativity and fear weaken it. Lasting unhappiness or a traumatic event can overwhelm our cells. It is no exaggeration to claim that our every thought and emotion equals a biochemical act. In the words of neuroscientist Dr Candace Pelt co-discoverer of endorphins, "Cells are conscious beings that communicate with each other, affecting our emotions and choices." It is equally true that our emotions and beliefs affect the activity of our cells.

Clearly, the patient's emotional health is of vital importance if we want to ensure that the Gerson Therapy brings optimum results.

Any cancer diagnosis equals a major trauma. It evokes powerful emotions: panic, fear, rage, or, at the opposite pole, resignation, numbness, despair. Either way, most patients experience a sense of isolation, of being cast out of normal life and deprived of a future. Harrowing memories of personally known cancer victims arise - contributing to a superstitious fear of the disease.

This fear springs from two sources. One is rational, based on the very real threat of suffering, disfigurement, drastic treatments with vile side elects, and probably no cure in the end. But there is a non-rational fear, too, which sees cancer as an intruder, an evil alien that has breached our defenses and may kill us. In their panic-stricken state very few patients realize that tumors don't come from outer space but from the faulty functioning of their own bodies. All these emotions are negative - heavy, distressing. And they are made worse by the average physician's response which is normally defensive and reserved, if not downright cold. (it was certainly cold in my experience when I presented with a secondary tumor and my previously friendly surgeon-oncologist suddenly turned icy, implying with his manner that by producing a lump in my groin I had somehow let the side down.)

If the patient then spends time in an average hospital, the additional handicap of dependence, loss of adult autonomy and privacy will make things even worse. The patient becomes a massive sufferer, with no say in what is being done to him or her. In the telling phrase of Ivan Illich, "Modern medicine turns the patient into a limp and mystified voyeur in the grip of bio-engineers."

These observations apply to cancer patients diagnosed and treated in an orthodox medical framework. But as almost all patients come to the Gerson Therapy from that system we must recognize their depressed, fearful or numb state and do something about it - fast. Ordinarily, humanity demands that we try to relieve their sense of isolation, fear and hopelessness, by giving them time, space and permission to unload their huge emotional burden.

But beside ordinary humanity, in the light of PNI's findings there are also sound medical reasons for urgently re-programming the patients' inner state from negative to positive. "No attempt should be made to cure the body without the soul," wrote the Greek philosopher Plato nearly 2400 years ago. In today's terms, even the brilliant Gerson program cannot do its best if something deep down in the patient's consciousness keeps saying "No" to life.

And that something may be a totally separate diagnosis. It may have to do with what Lawrence LeShan, pioneer researcher of the body-mind link in malignant disease, dubbed "the cancer-prone personality". Other researchers soon confirmed his observation that certain personality traits seemed to pre-dispose some people to cancer. In LeShan's formulation, these traits include low self-esteem, difficulty in expressing anger or aggression, a tendency to please others and ignore his/her own needs and feelings. In other words, the true self of such a person has disappeared behind a false self, developed probably in early childhood and maintained in adulthood, although no longer necessary.

Naturally, this personality profile is only a model and does not apply to all cancer patients, although in my work with sufferers over nearly fourteen years I have often come across these character traits. What matters is that - together or separately - they signal a negative outlook on life which a cancer diagnosis can turn into bleak despair; and PNI tells us clearly what that means in trends of reduced immune competence.

It is well known that cancer often appears 18 months or two years after some untoward life event, such as bereavement, divorce, career crisis, fiscal blow, and so on. Experience with clients has shown me that those events only represented the last straw that ultimately broke the camel's back; that, indeed, those people had long existed in what they had felt was a life trap, an impossible existential situation that apparently could neither be borne nor changed. LeShan and Carl Simonton, M.D., describe this life trap in detail. My own case material bears out its existence, and also the fact that those who feel unable to escape eventually reach a stage when they don't care whether they live or die. As many of them have told me, "Something snapped." I suspect it was the last strand of their will to live.

And, as the well-known saying has it, "Cancer is a socially acceptable form of suicide."

What we are dealing with here is the mysterious interaction of biochemist and emotions, a vast new area of body-mind medicine which we are only beginning to explore. But there is already enough orthodox clinical, as opposed to anecdotal, evidence to prove that inner attitudes can make a big difference to survival.

In a now classical study, British researcher Stephen Greer interviewed a group of women three months after they had undergone mastectomies, to find out how they were coping. He found four distinct types among them who showed, respectively, fighting spirit, denial, stoic acceptance, and hopelessness. After 5 and 10 years, 80% of the fighters, but only 20% of the hopeless had survived. These rates had nothing to do with medical prognoses.

In the U.S., David Spiegel, M.D., of Stanford, invited a group of 56 women with metastasized breast cancer to attend weekly meetings for a year, where they could share worries and sorrows, encourage each ether, and change their mental attitude. A control group of 50 women attended no such meetings. Spiegel only wanted to discover whether the group activity enhanced the members' quality of life, which it certainly did. But, to his amazement, he found that they also lived twice as long as those that did not attend.

These studies, as well as my own case histories suggest that the fighters, unlike the despondent patients, give positive non-verbal messages to their bodies which boost their immune system, and get results accordingly. Not always. Humanity's mortality rate remains obstinately 100%, but we don't all have to go at once.

Still, on the orthodox side, an interesting insight comes from U.S. oncologist-surgeon Bernie Siegal, M.D., author of several best-selling books which have helped to extend public understanding of the body-mind link in health and sickness. He claims that 15-20% of cancer patients unconsciously or consciously want to die, no doubt to get out of a bad life trap. 60-70% wish to get well but are passive and expect the doctor to do all the work. 15-20%, however, are exceptional: they refuse to play victim, they research their disease, don't obey the doctor automatically but ask questions, demand control and make informed choices. In Bernie Siegel's words, "Difficult or uncooperative patients are most likely to get well. " Apparently they have more killer T-cells than docile patients. I suspect that many Gerson patients would qualify for membership in Bernie Siegel's groups of Exceptional Cancer Patients.

So how do we go about promoting a positive outlook and a fighting spirit in the patient?

The best I can offer is what I have learned and practiced over the years. The following steps refer to all patients with cancer or other chronic degenerative diseases; the specific needs of Gerson patients will be discussed afterwards. The first step is to de-mystify the disease, discuss it openly, in a natural voice, without euphemisms or technical jargon. This helps to provide a safe space where the patient can find emotional release, encouraged by being listened to with total, non-judgmental attention.

I always ask the initial question, "Do you want to live?" If the answer is yes, I ask, "Do you want to live unconditionally?" Another firm "yes" settles that matter. But often a "yes, but..." reply identifies an undecided individual, and the need for further exploration.

It is important to build a therapeutic partnership with the patient and give him or her responsibility and an active role to play. We must be totally honest, have the courage to say "I don't know" when we don't refuse any kind of prognosis. If a patient tells us that 85% of people with his condition die within three years, we invite him to join the 15% who don't. (I recall with joy and admiration the fragile little lady riddled with cancer who, when told that she had six months to live, brightly replied, "Oh good, I have six months to get well." And get well she did, on the Gerson Therapy...)

The 18-24 months of the patient's life prior to the diagnosis can yield valuable clues. Did some major stress drive the patient to drink, drugs or other destructive habits which caused significant liver damage? Gentle questioning often allows us to identify some life trap; the next task is to show that there is a way out, other than dying.

To flush out the inner saboteur, we need to help the patient recognize and release self-defeating patterns, old unfinished business, and resentment - especially resentment, since the repeated reliving of old hurts, rage or pain puts the autonomic nervous system into distress mode, which is the last thing the patient needs.

Reprogramming means shifting the emphasis from negative to positive. To quote LeShan once again, his basic question is "What's right with you?" What are your special ways of being, relating, creating? What is blocking their expression? What do you need to fulfill yourself? Above all, what do YOU want to do with your life?"

I agree with LeShan's claim that under the circumstances it is permissible to ask questions which one would avoid otherwise. Questions like: If you had another thirty years to live, would you remarry your spouse? or stay with your partner? or remain in your present career?

Once these important basics have been clarified, it is time to switch from the passive to the active mode and point out the enormous potential open to the patient, if only he or she will act, not just react, and start making personal decisions. After all, there is nothing to lose.

If possible, the family dynamics should also be explored. A toxic relationship - to a spouse, an over-demanding parent or antagonistic children - may contribute to the disease. Without recognizing the situation there is no way to ease it.

A great deal can be achieved in a short time. The main tool of the physician or therapist is his or her personality and calm, reliable presence. Often this presence is the only solid support to the patient's confused, chaotic world. Other tools, such as teaching relaxation techniques, simple meditation, and creative visualization, focused on self-healing, can and should he used later, by suitably trained counselors and therapists.

Beside the trauma and psychological needs experienced by cancer sufferers in general, Gerson patients have extra burdens to bear. Far too many come to the therapy as a last resort, after conventional treatments have failed them, leaving behind a sense of disappointment, betrayal, and a range of severe after-effects. For them, embarking on the Gerson Therapy is like taking a mad gamble, an end-of-the-line decision.

Others choose the Gerson path at an earlier, less serious stage of their disease, with fewer preventable changes in their bodies, but with a poor prognosis.

Either way they embark on an unfamiliar treatment, much of which sounds bizarre at first.

They step outside the boundaries of orthodox medicine, the network of doctors, consultants, hospitals, referrals; a whole system which has been unable to heal them yet still carries an aura of great power. Some may have been shown the door by their physician. Others face pressure and doubts from family members and friends who don't see how a weird, never-heard-of therapy can succeed where modern high-tech medicine has failed.

The would-be patient's own doubts spring largely from the sheer length of the therapy. In the more familiar allopathic field of medicine there is a pill for every ill, you either recover or you die, but at least things happen fast. To face two years of unremitting effort, strict discipline and monotony sounds pretty horrendous, especially because there is no guarantee of success at the other end. This explains why only a small percentage of inquirers chooses to embark on the therapy (in the U.K. the uptake is around 20%) after digesting the first batch of information.

We can assume a certain toughness and determination, or sheer despair, in those who are willing to make a start. At this stage, their main need is for reassurance, for sober hope mixed with honest realism. They need to hear that theirs is a serious disease indeed, but it is possible to recover from it, and the Gerson Therapy is the most logical way to regain their health. This is when the cognitive approach works best, explaining the "how" and the "why" of the Gerson program. It needs no medical background to understand why rebuilding the immune system is a better idea than knocking it out with radiation and a cocktail of toxic substances.

And so, by this stage having settled the emotional overload of the patient, we work along rational lines, explaining, answering questions, not asking anything to be taken on trust. This reinforces the patient's involvement in the healing process as an equal partner and ally of the doctor or specialist counselor.

To get an overview, it helps to imagine the two or more years of the Gerson Therapy as a drama in three acts.

Act One

Starting out. A time of excitement and exploration, unfamiliarity, drastic changes in lifestyle, diet, daily routine. Much to learn all the time. It is a great advantage to start the therapy at a Gerson clinic. But, sooner or later, there follows the expulsion from that Garden of Eden where everything is done for the patient, and reality must be faced at home. For the patient who starts at home, chaos sets in - temporarily from Day One.

At first, the sheer tasks of the day seem impossible: preparing juices, food, enema coffee, washing up endlessly, securing deliveries, checking on the helper, cleaning up after the helper - above all, remaining sane. At this stage, practical help is essential almost round the clock, to stop the patient from giving up at once.

Act One is so busy and active that there is little space and time for psychological matters.

Act Two

The main part (possibly the longest second act on Earth). The daily routine has been established and is rolling along, but even with helpers it demands time, effort and perseverance. The monotony and boredom begin to tell on the patient who feels restricted, under virtual house arrest. In theory it is possible to go out after dinner, in practice it does not happen often.

Then there is the problem of flare-ups or healing reactions which can be vile yet have to be welcomed, since they signal that the body is responding to the therapy. By way of psychological support the reasons and symptoms of flare-ups must be explained in advance, so that the patient does not panic (while feeling terrible). "This, too, will pass" is the best comfort we can offer.

An opposite problem, admittedly much rarer, is when there are no flare-ups for a while, and the patient immediately concludes that the therapy is not working, there is no hope left. I remember my own despondency all those years ago when, except for one almighty flare-up, I did not have any for months. It really worried me. Then I had twenty-six in a row, which gave me something else to worry about.

Physical detoxification inevitably brings about psychological detoxification, too. Toxins passing through the central nervous system evoke strange reactions and out-of-character behavior: violent mood swings, snappiness, anger, instability, unfair accusations and aggression. The patient's normally civilized behavior gives way to drives and emotions that have been denied and repressed for a long time, perhaps since childhood. The adult "censor" within is pushed aside by a raging infant, at least for a while, and then takes over again, amidst profuse apologies.

This, too, has to be prepared for, and not taken personally; it is part of the process. In whatever capacity we work with the patient, we remain calm, caring, unchanged, waiting for the inner upheaval to pass.

However, we need to be more active if depression sets in. This, too, can be the result of the detoxification process, or of some small adverse symptom which is immediately seen as ominous. A bad result in the latest blood test or an apparent change in a palpable tumor can plunge the patient into black despair. This has to be dispelled fast by pointing out that there are many ups and downs and fluctuations within the healing process, so that single symptoms are not signals of doom.

Depression can also set in when the patient gets terminally fed up and wants to quit the therapy, although improvements are noticeable. It is best not to contradict the patient's grumbles but, on the contrary, agree that the process is demanding, monotonous, restricting and boring; and then point out the good results so far, ask tactless questions, such as, "Would you rather have chemotherapy?" or "All right, you give up - and then what?" and wait for the answer.

Remember: this, too, will pass.

Taking life day by day, one day at a tine, is a good way to handle the apparent endlessness of the therapy, without losing sight of the ultimate aim. In fact, interim goal-setting - what would the patient want to achieve in one week, one month and three months - helps even further to break up the monotony. The aims should be realistic and modest, and warmly acknowledged when they are achieved. Those that did not work out can be rephrased or postponed but not written off as failures.

Food can be a major issue during the main part of the therapy. Many people take to Gerson food at once and enjoy it. Others do not. When resistance wells up and turns mealtimes into the adult equivalent of nursery tantrums, we are up against the deep emotional investment many people have in certain types of food, however unhealthy. Their attachment is probably to the food mother gave then in childhood when food equaled love, even if it was low-grade junk. At a fraught time such people may feel that what they eat is their last area of free choice, and even though on a mental level they accept the rightness of the Gerson diet, on a deeper non-rational level they reject it, sometimes literally.

This is where wise counseling is needed. The patient must be reminded that the food on offer is medicine, that the diet is not for ever, and that accepting it now is a sound investment in the future. I have found it helpful to make a solemn contract with the patient who undertook to stick to the diet meticulously for a fortnight. As a rule, quick improvement followed and extending the contract proved easy.

The need to observe the rules cannot be overstated. Small lapses and occasional exceptions, often asked for by patients, are out of the question, for what exactly is small, and how often does an occasional exception occur? Once the rules are broken, the safe boundaries of the therapy are damaged, and the consequences can be serious. However, as carers or therapists we must enforce the rules with tact and affection, otherwise we may end up in the role of the overstrict parent, with "Thou shalt not" written all over us.

During the long main part of the therapy, the patient's boredom can be relieved by providing relevant reading material and tapes, set up networking with other Gerson Persons, or encourage a fresh hobby or study that can be fitted in between juices, enemas and meals. Friends' behavior can be crucial. Can they bear the patient's illness and face their own fears, or do they fade out of the picture? And how are the family members coping? Are they bearing the burden of the therapy without making the patient feel guilty?

Act Three

Winding down. The intensive therapy is over. Now is the time to taper it off more and more, cutting down gradually on juices, enemas, medication, preparing to re-enter the world.

This can be a very tricky phase. The same patients who used to ask, "Is there life after Gerson?" now are reluctant to let go of the routine. It has become a way of life which has served them superbly. They feel and look well, they are symptom-free, with good test results and no complaints. But they do not want to come off the therapy.

By then it has become their safety device and symbolic life-and-health insurance, with the implied fear that stopping the therapy may bring on a relapse. This fear must not be dismissed lightly: it requires a careful, patient "weaning process" to ensure that the tube of the enema bucket does not turn into a substitute umbilical cord. Sticking with the dietary principles set out by Dr. Gerson is very necessary for the rest of one's life, in order to safeguard one's bravely rebuilt health.

There are others, of course, who have to be restrained from rushing back into their erstwhile disastrous eating habits at the end of Act Three. As a rule, the attempt is doomed: their detoxified, cleared, optimally nourished systems tend to shrink away from so-called normal food, heavy with fat and painfully salty. If their understanding does not object to junk food, their taste buds will.

In my experience, after recovery there is no way back into the pre-disease state. The experience of the holistic Gerson Therapy changes you, not only in your lifestyle and eating habits but also in your value system, priorities and general outlook. You have been reborn without the need to die first, and you may easily and naturally decide to help others, by way of repaying a debt to life.

Appendix I: Lab Tests

Laboratory testing of blood and urine are a standard part of your Gerson physician's follow-up protocol for Gerson Therapy patients. The following compendium of explanations and interpretations is provided to help people feel less intimidated by unfamiliar terms, and to acquaint them with current knowledge.

Either *Gould's Medical Dictionary* or *Taber's Cyclopedic Medical Dictionary* will prove an indispensable aid. Also valuable will be the *Webster's Unabridged International Dictionary* (published by Merriam Co.).

One of the first realizations the reader will have is that lab values shift frequently, rapidly, and for a wide variety of reasons. Even large shifts which fall within or close to normal indicated limits should not be cause for alarm. Results of a single set of chemistries or counts are never conclusive. Remarkable results, those which fall far outside of normal limits, warrant retesting and future monitoring.

The following laboratory test report is an example taken from the chart of a Gerson patient. Headings below are number-referenced to this report. Please note that no two laboratories use the same forms or necessarily group tests in the same way. Although most labs are now using standardized reporting systems, some labs will use ranges of findings which differ from those below.

PATIENT NAME					PATIENT ID.				SPEC. NO		SPEC. DATE	
BONE		**ELECTROLYTES**			**HEART**		**LIVER**				**LIPIDS**	
Calcium mg/dl (8.5-10.5) **1.**	Phosphorous mg/dl (2.5-4.5) **2.**	Sodium mEq/L (135-148) **3.**	Potassium mEq/L (3.5-5.5) **4.**	Chloride mEq/L (95-110) **5.**	LDH IU/L (90-225) **6.**	AST (SGOT) IU/L (3-45) **7.**	T. Bili mg/dl (3-45) **8.**	GGT (IU/L) (M 2-65) (F 2-45) **9.**	ALT (SGPT) IU/L (3-50) **10.**	Alk. Phos. IU/L (30-128) **11.**	Cholesterol mg/dl <200 **12.**	Triglycerides mg/dl (35-200) **13.**
PROTEIN				**KIDNEY**		**THYROID**				**MISCELLANEOUS**		
T Protein g/dl (6.0-8.0) **14.**	Globulin g/dl (2.0-4.0) **15.**	Albumin g/dl (3.5-5.0) **16.**	A/G Ratio (1.0-2.5) **17.**	BUN mg/dl (6-25) **18.**	Creatinine mg/dl (0.6-1.5) **19.**	T_4 µg/dl (4.5-12.5)	T_3 Uptake % (33-45)	Free T_4 Index (1.5-5.6)	TSH µ IU/L (0.3-5.9)	Uric Acid mg/dl (M 3.0-9.0) (F 2.2-7.7) **20.**	Glucose mg/dl <50 yrs. (70-110) **21.**	Iron ug/dl (35-180) **22.**
						Thyroid tests not reliable when iodine (Lugol's) and Thyroid hormone are given.						

HEMATOLOGY														
RBC $\times 10^6$/mm^3 (M 4.3-5.9) (F 3.5-5.5) **23.**	HGB g/dl (M 13.9-18.0) (F 12.0-16.0) **24.**	HCT % (M 39-55) (F 36-48) **25.**	MCV µ3 (80-100) **26.**	MCH µµg (26-34) **27.**	MCHC % (31-37) **28.**	Platelets x 10^3/mm^3 (140-440) **29.**	WBC x 10^3/mm^3 (4.0-10.5) **30.**	Polys (45-75%) (1.5-8.0)	Bands (0-5%)	Metas (0%)	Lymphs (20-45%) (0.8-3.2)	Mono (0-10%) (0.0-0.8)	EOS (0-6%) (0-0.5)	BASO (0-2%) (0-0.1)
										(See WBC differential) % ABSOLUTE VALUES				

RESULTS ARE FLAGGED IN ACCORDANCE WITH AGE DEPENDENT REFERENCE RANGES WHICH ARE SUMMARIZED ON THE BACK OF THIS REPORT.

*** A comment applied to this test has been printed in the body of the report.**

1. Calcium, serum

This test measures serum levels of calcium, a predominantly extracellular cation that helps regulate and promote neuromuscular and enzyme activity, skeletal development, and blood coagulation. The body absorbs calcium from the gastrointestinal tract, provided sufficient vitamin D is present, and excretes it in the urine and feces. Over 98% of the body's calcium can shift in and out of these structures. For example, when calcium concentrations in the blood fall below normal, calcium ions can move out of the bones and teeth to help restore blood levels.

Parathyroid hormone, vitamin D, and to a lesser extent, calcitonin and adrenal steroids control calcium blood levels. Calcium and phosphorus are closely related, usually reacting together to form insoluble calcium phosphate. To prevent formation of a precipitate in the blood, calcium levels vary inversely with phosphorus; as serum calcium levels rise, phosphorus levels should decrease through renal excretion. Since the body excretes calcium daily, regular ingestion of calcium in food (at least 1 g/day) is necessary for normal calcium balance.

Purpose

To aid diagnosis of neuromuscular, skeletal, and endocrine disorders; arrhythmias; blood-clotting deficiencies; and acid-base imbalance.

Values

Normally, serum calcium levels range from 8.9 to 10.1 mg/dl (atomic absorption; 2.25 to 2.75 mmol/L). In children, serum calcium levels are higher than in adults. Calcium levels can rise as high as 12 mg/dl (3.0 mmol/L) during phases of rapid bone growth.

Implications of results

Abnormally high serum calcium levels (hypercalcemia) may occur in hyperparathyroidism and parathyroid tumors (caused by oversecretion of parathyroid hormone), Paget's disease of the bone, multiple myeloma, metastatic carcinoma, multiple fractures, or prolonged immobilization. Elevated serum calcium levels may also result from inadequate excretion of calcium, as in adrenal insufficiency and renal disease; from excessive calcium ingestion; or from overuse of antacids such as calcium carbonate.

Low calcium levels (hypocalcemia) may result from hypoparathyroidism, total parathyroidectomy, or malabsorption. Decreased serum levels of calcium may follow calcium loss in Cushing's syndrome, renal failure, acute pancreatitis, and peritonitis.

Clinical Alert: Observe the patient with hypercalcemia for deep bone pain, flank pain caused by renal calculi, and muscle hypotonicity. Hypercalcemic crisis begins with nausea, vomiting, and dehydration, leading to stupor and coma, and can end in cardiac arrest.

In a patient with hypocalcemia, be alert for circumoral and peripheral numbness and tingling, muscle twitching, Chvostek's sign (facial muscle spasm), tetany, muscle cramping. Trousseau's sign (carpopedal spasm), seizures, and arrhythmias.

2. Phosphates, serum

This test measures serum levels of phosphates, the dominant cellular anions. Phosphates help store and utilize body energy, and help regulate calcium levels, carbohydrate and lipid metabolism, and acid-base balance. Phosphates are essential to bone formation; about 85% of the body's phosphates are found in bone. The intestine absorbs a considerable amount of phosphates from dietary sources, but adequate levels of vitamin D are necessary for their absorption. The kidneys excrete phosphates and serve as a regulatory mechanism. Because calcium and phosphate interact in a reciprocal relationship, urinary excretion of phosphates increases or decreases in inverse proportion to serum calcium levels. Abnormal concentrations of phosphates result more often from improper excretion than from abnormal ingestion or absorption from dietary sources.

Purpose

- To aid diagnosis of renal disorders and acid-base imbalance.
- To detect endocrine, skeletal, and calcium disorders.

Values

Normally, serum phosphate levels range from 2.5 to 4.5 mg/dl (0.80 to 1.40 mmol/L) or from 1.8 to 2.6 mEq/liter. Children have higher serum phosphate levels than adults. Phosphate levels can rise as high as 7 mg/dl (2.25 mmol/L) during periods of increased bone growth.

Implications of results

Because serum phosphate values alone are of limited use diagnostically (only a few rare conditions directly affect phosphate metabolism), they should be interpreted in light of serum calcium results.

Depressed phosphate levels (hypophosphatemia) may result from malnutrition, malabsorption syndromes, hyperparathyroidism, renal tubular acidosis, or treatment of diabetic acidosis. In children, hypophosphatemia can suppress normal growth.

Elevated levels (hyperphosphatemia) may result from skeletal disease, healing fractures, hypoparathyroidism, acromegaly, diabetic acidosis, high intestinal obstruction, and renal failure. Hyperphosphatemia is rarely clinically significant; however, if prolonged, it can alter bone metabolism by causing abnormal calcium phosphate deposits.

3. Sodium, serum

This test measures serum levels of sodium, the major extracellular cation. Sodium affects body water distribution, maintains osmotic pressure of extracellular fluid, and helps promote neuromuscular function; it also helps maintain acid-base balance and influences chloride and potassium levels. Sodium is absorbed by the intestines and is excreted primarily by the kidneys; a small amount is lost through the skin.

Since extracellular sodium concentration helps the kidneys to regulate body water (decreased sodium levels promote water excretion and increased levels promote retention), serum levels of sodium are evaluated in relation to the amount of water in the body. For example, a sodium deficit (hyponatremia) refers to a decreased level of sodium in relation to the body's water level. The body normally regulates this sodium-water balance through aldosterone, which inhibits sodium excretion and promotes its resorption (with water) by the renal tubules, to maintain balance. Low sodium levels stimulate aldosterone secretion; elevated sodium levels depress aldosterone secretion.

Special Note: *In the context of the Gerson Therapy, both sodium and chloride levels may occasionally fall below normal limits for the general population. When this occurs, frequent monitoring of electrolytes and continuous clinical observation are warranted. In most cases, sodium spilling is self-limiting. Reduction of edema through elimination of sodium is the goal of sodium restriction and potassium supplementation. The body mechanisms which are accelerated by the Gerson Therapy in order to remove sodium from diseased tissue will not normally cause a severe reduction of serum sodium which is essential for life.* ***Note:*** *When below normal sodium levels occur, the Gerson physician should be immediately consulted.*

Purpose

- To evaluate fluid-electrolyte and acid-base balance, and related neuromuscular, renal, and adrenal functions.
- To evaluate the effects of drug therapy (such as diuretics) on serum sodium levels.

Values

Normally serum sodium levels range from 135 to 145 mEq/liter (mmol/L).

Implications of results

Sodium imbalance can result from a loss or gain of sodium, or from a change in water volume. Serum sodium results must be interpreted in light of the patient's state of hydration.

Elevated serum sodium levels (hypernatremia) may be caused by inadequate water intake, water loss in excess of sodium (as in diabetes insipidus, impaired renal function, prolonged hyperventilation, and occasionally, severe vomiting or diarrhea), and sodium retention (as in aldosteronism). Hypernatremia can also result from excessive sodium intake.

Clinical Alert: In a patient with hypernatremia and associated loss of water, observe for signs of thirst, restlessness, dry and sticky mucous membranes, flushed skin, oliguria, and diminished reflexes. However, if increased total body sodium causes water retention, observe for hypertension, dyspnea, and edema.

Abnormally low serum sodium levels (hyponatremia) may result from inadequate sodium intake or excessive sodium loss caused by profuse sweating, gastrointestinal suctioning. diuretic therapy, diarrhea, vomiting, adrenal insufficiency, burns, or chronic renal insufficiency with acidosis. Urine sodium determinations are frequently more sensitive to early changes in sodium balance and should always be evaluated simultaneously with serum sodium findings.

In a patient with hyponatremia, watch for apprehension, lassitude, headache, decreased skin turgor, abdominal cramps, and tremors that may progress to convulsions.

4. Potassium, serum

This test, a quantitative analysis, measures serum levels of potassium, the major intracellular cation. Small amounts of potassium may also be found in extracellular fluid. Vital to homeostasis, potassium maintains cellular osmotic equilibrium and helps regulate muscle activity (it's essential in maintaining electrical conduction within the cardiac and skeletal muscles). Potassium also helps regulate enzyme activity and acid-base balance, and influences kidney function. Potassium levels are affected by variations in the secretion of adrenal steroid hormones, and by fluctuations in pH, serum glucose levels, and serum sodium levels. A reciprocal relationship appears to exist between potassium and sodium; a substantial intake of one element causes a corresponding decrease in the other. Although it readily conserves sodium, the body has no efficient method for conserving potassium. Even in potassium depletion, the kidneys continue to excrete potassium; therefore, potassium deficiency can develop rapidly and is quite common.

Since the kidneys excrete nearly all the ingested potassium, a dietary intake of at least 40 mEq/day (mmol/d) is essential. (A normal diet usually includes 60 to 100 mEq [mmol/d] potassium.)

Purpose

• To evaluate clinical signs of potassium excess (hyperkalemia) or potassium depletion (hypokalemia).

• To monitor renal function, acid-base balance, and glucose metabolism.

• To evaluate neuromuscular and endocrine disorders.

• To detect the origin of arrhythmias.

Values

Normally, serum potassium levels range from 3.8 to 5.5 mEq/liter (mmol/L).

Implications of results

Abnormally high serum potassium levels (hyperkalemia) are common in patients with bums, crushing injuries, diabetic ketoacidosis, and myocardial infarction - conditions in which excessive cellular potassium enters the blood. Hyperkalemia may also indicate reduced sodium excretion, possibly because of renal failure (preventing normal sodium-potassium exchange) or Addison's disease (caused by the absence of aldosterone, with consequent potassium buildup and sodium depletion).

Note: *Although elevated serum potassium is uncommon in Gerson patients, if it does occur, supplemental potassium should be discontinued and the Gerson physician should be immediately consulted.*

Clinical Alert: Observe a patient with hyperkalemia for weakness, malaise, nausea, diarrhea, colicky pain, muscle irritability progressing to flaccid paralysis, oliguria, and bradycardia. Electrocardiogram (ECG) reveals a prolonged PR interval; wide QRS; tall, tented T wave; and ST depression.

Below-normal potassium values often result from aldosteronism or Cushing's syndrome (marked by hypersecretion of adrenal steroid hormones), loss of body fluids (as in long-term diuretic therapy), or excessive licorice ingestion (because of the aldosterone-like effect of glycyrrhizic acid). Although serum values and clinical symptoms can indicate a potassium imbalance, an ECG provides the definitive diagnosis.

Clinical Alert (2): Observe a patient with hypokalemia for decreased reflexes; rapid, weak, irregular pulse; mental confusion; hypotension; anorexia; muscle weakness; and paresthesia. ECG shows a flattened T wave, ST depression, and U wave elevation. In severe cases. ventricular fibrillation, respiratory paralysis, and cardiac arrest can develop.

Interfering factors

Excessive or rapid potassium infusion, spironolactone or penicillin G potassium therapy, or renal toxicity from administration of amphotericin B, methicillin, or tetracycline increases serum potassium levels.

Insulin and glucose administration, diuretic therapy (especially with thiazides, but not with triamterene, amiloride, or spironolactone), or I.V. infusions without potassium decrease serum potassium levels.

Excessive hemolysis of the sample or delay in drawing blood following application of a tourniquet increases potassium levels.

5. Chloride, serum

This test, a quantitative analysis, measures serum levels of chloride, the major extracellular fluid anion. Interacting with sodium, chloride helps maintain the osmotic pressure of blood and therefore helps regulate blood volume and arterial pressure. Chloride levels also affect acid-base balance. Serum concentrations of this electrolyte are regulated by aldosterone secondarily to regulation of sodium. Chloride is absorbed from the intestines and is excreted primarily by the kidneys.

Purpose

• To detect acid-base imbalance (acidosis and alkalosis) and to aid evaluation of fluid status and extracellular cation-anion balance.

Values

Normally serum chloride levels range from 100 to 108 mEq/liter (mmol/L).

Implications of results

Chloride levels relate inversely to those of bicarbonate and thus reflect acid-base balance. Excessive loss of gastric juices or of other secretions containing chloride may cause hypochloremic metabolic alkalosis; excessive chloride retention or ingestion may lead to hyperchloremic metabolic acidosis.

Elevated serum chloride levels (hypercloremia) may result from severe dehydration, complete renal shutdown, head injury (producing neurogenic hyperventilation), and primary aldosteronism.

Low chloride levels (hypochloremia) are usually associated with low sodium and potassium levels. Possible underlying causes include prolonged vomiting, gastric suctioning, intestinal fistula, chronic renal failure, and Addison's disease. Congestive heart failure, or edema resulting in excess extracellular fluid can cause dilutional hypochloremia. Note: If below normal chloride levels occur, the Gerson physician should be immediately consulted.

Clinical Alert: Observe a patient with hypochloremia for hypertonicity of muscles, tetany, and depressed respirations. In a patient with hyperchloremia, be alert for signs of developing stupor, rapid deep breathing, and weakness that may lead to coma.

6. Lactic dehydrogenase (LDH)

Lactic dehydrogenase (LDH) is an enzyme that catalyzes the reversible conversion of muscle pyruvic acid into lactic acid. Because LDH is present in almost all body tissues, cellular damage causes an elevation of total serum LDH, thus limiting the diagnostic usefulness of LDH. However, five tissue specific isoenzymes can be identified and measured, using heat inactivation or electrophoresis: two of these isoenzymes, LDH(I) and LDH(2), appear primarily in the heart, red blood cells, and kidneys; LDH(3), primarily in the lungs; and LDH(4) and LDH(5), in the liver and the skeletal muscles.

The specificity of LDH isoenzymes and their distribution pattern is useful in diagnosing hepatic, pulmonary, and erythrocytic damage. But its widest clinical application (with other cardiac enzyme tests) is in diagnosing acute myocardial infarction (MI). LDH isoenzyme assay is also useful when creatine phosphokinase (CPK) hasn't been measured within 24 hours of an acute MI. The myocardial LDH level rises later than CPK (12 to 48 hours after infarction begins), peaks in 2 to 5 days, and drops to normal in 7 to 10 days, if tissue necrosis doesn't persist.

Purpose

• To aid differential diagnosis of MI, pulmonary infarction, anemias, and hepatic disease.

• To support CPK isoenzyme test results in diagnosing MI, or to provide diagnosis when CPK-MB samples are drawn too late to display elevation.

• To monitor patient response to some forms of chemotherapy.

Values

Total LDH levels normally range from 48 to 115 U/L. Normal distribution is as follows -

LDH(I): 17.5% to 28.3% of total
LDH(2): 30.4% to 36.4% of total
LDH(3): 19.2% to 24.8% of total
LDH(4): 9.6% to 15.6% of total
LDH(5): 5.5% to 12.7% of total

Implications of results

Since many common diseases cause elevations in total LDH levels, isoenzymeelectrophoresis is usually necessary for diagnosis. In some disorders, total LDH may be within normal limits, but abnormal proportions of each enzyme indicate specific organ tissue damage. For instance, in acute MI, the concentration of LDH(I) is greater than LDH(2) within 12 to 48 hours after onset of symptoms. This reversal of normal isoenzyme patterns is typical of myocardial damage and is referred to as flipped LDH.

7. SGOT / AST

(Aspartate transaminase, serum: glutamic-oxaloacetic transaminase, serum

Aspartate aminotransferase (AST), is one of two enzymes that catalyze the transfer of the nitrogenous portion of amino acid to an amino acid residue. AST is found in the cytoplasm and mitochondria of many cells, primarily in the liver, heart, skeletal muscles, kidneys, pancreas, and to a lesser extent, in red blood cells. It is released into serum in proportion to cellular damage.

Although a high correlation

exists between myocardial infarction (MI) and elevated AST, this test is sometimes considered superfluous for diagnosing MI because of its relatively low organ specificity; it doesn't enable differentiation between acute MI and the effects of hepatic congestion due to heart failure.

Purpose

• To detect recent MI (together with creatine phosphokinase and lactate dehydrogenase).

• To aid detection and differential diagnosis of acute hepatic disease.

• To monitor patient progress and prognosis in cardiac and hepatic diseases.

Values

AST levels by a commonly used method range from 8 to 20 U/L. Normal values for infants are as high as four times those of adults.

Implications of results

AST levels fluctuate in response to the extent of cellular necrosis and therefore may be transiently and minimally elevated early in the disease process, and extremely elevated during the most acute phase. Depending on when the initial sample was drawn, AST levels can rise - indicating increasing disease severity and tissue damage - or fall - indicating disease resolution and tissue repair. Thus, the relative change in AST values serves as a reliable monitoring mechanism.

Maximum elevations are associated with certain diseases and conditions. For example, very high elevations (more than 20 times normal) may indicate acute viral hepatitis, severe skeletal muscle trauma, extensive surgery, drug-induced hepatic injury, and severe passive liver congestion.

High levels: (ranging from 10 to 20 times normal) may indicate severe myocardial infarction, severe infectious mononucleosis, and alcoholic cirrhosis. High levels may also occur during the prodromal or resolving stages of conditions that cause maximal elevations.

Moderate-to-high levels: (ranging from 5 to 10 times normal) may indicate Duchennne muscular dystrophy, dermatomyositis, and chronic hepatitis. Moderate-to-high levels also occur during prodromal and resolving stages of diseases that cause high elevations.

Low-to-moderate levels: (ranging from 2 to 5 times normal) may indicate hemolytic anemia, metastatic hepatic tumors, acute pancreatitis, pulmonary emboli, alcohol withdrawal syndrome, and fatty liver. AST levels rise slightly after the first few days of biliary duct obstruction. Also, low-to-moderate elevations occur at some time during any of the preceding conditions or diseases.

8. Bilirubin, serum

This test measures serum levels of bilirubin, the predominant pigment in bile. Bilirubin is the major product of hemoglobin catabolism. After being formed in the reticuloendothelial cells, bilirubin is bound to albumin and is transported to the liver, where it is conjugated with glucuronic acid to form bilirubin glucuronide and bilirubin diglucuronide - compounds that are then excreted in bile.

Effective conjugation and excretion of bilirubin depends on a properly functioning hepatobiliary system and a normal red blood cell turnover rate. Therefore, measurement of unconjugated (indirect or prehepatic) bilirubin, and conjugated (direct or posthepatic) bilirubin can help evaluate hepatobiliary and erythropoietic functions. Serum bilirubin measurements are especially significant in neonates because elevated unconjugated bilirubin can accumulate in the brain (kernicterus) and cause irreparable tissue damage.

Elevated indirect serum bilirubin levels often indicate hepatic damage in which the parenchymal calls can no longer conjugate bilirubin with glucuronide. Consequently, indirect bilirubin reenters the bloodstream. High levels of indirect bilirubin are also likely in severe hemolytic anemia, when excessive indirect bilirubin overwhelms the liver's conjugating mechanism. If hemolysis continues, both direct and indirect bilirubin may rise.

Purpose

• To evaluate liver function.

• To aid differential diagnosis of jaundice and to monitor the progression of this disorder.

• To aid diagnosis of biliary obstruction and hemolytic anemia.

• To determine whether a neonate requires an exchange transfusion or phototherapy because of dangerously high levels of unconjugated bilirubin.

Values

Normally in an adult, indirect serum bilirubin measures I.I mg/dl or less; direct serum bilirubin, less than 0.5 mg/dl. Total serum bilirubin in neonates ranges from I to 12 mg/dl.

Implications of results

Elevated serum levels of indirect bilirubin indicate hemolysis (for example in G-6PD deficiency, autoimmunity, or transfusion reaction); hemolytic or pernicious anemia or hemorrhage; hepatocellular dysfunction (possibly resulting from viral hepatitis or congenital enzyme deficiencies, such as Gilbert's disease and Crigler-Najjar syndrome); or neonatal hepatic immaturity.

Elevated levels of direct conjugated bilirubin usually indicate biliary obstruction, in which direct bilirubin, blocked from its normal pathway from the liver into the biliary tree, overflows into the bloodstream. Biliary obstruction may be intrahepatic (viral hepatitis, cirrhosis, chlorpromazine reaction), extrahepatic (gallstones, gallbladder or pancreatic carcinoma), or result from bile duct disease. If biliary obstruction continues, both direct and indirect bilirubin may be eventually elevated because of hepatic damage. In severe chronic hepatic damage, direct bilirubin concentrations may return to normal or near-normal levels, but elevated indirect bilirubin levels persist.

In neonates, total bilirubin levels that reach or exceed 20 mg/dl indicate the need for exchange transfusion.

9. Gamma-glutamyl transpeptidase (GGT), serum

Gamma-glutamyl transpeptidase (GGT) is most commonly elevated in hepatobiliary disease. This enzyme is very sensitive to drug induction and, therefore, is often used to detect recent alcohol ingestion, which is important in determining compliance with treatment of alcoholism. GGT is more sensitive than alkaline phosphatase in predicting cholestatic processes and neoplastic liver disease. However, its sensitivity to induction by drugs is problematic in regard to specificity.

Purpose

- To aid diagnosis of obstructive jaundice in neoplastic liver disease and detection of recent alcohol consumption.
- When used with alkaline phosphatase, to suggest the source of elevated alkaline phosphatase levels.

Values

The normal range for GGT varies considerably with age in males but is not affected in females. The normal range in males between ages 18 to 50 is 10 to 39 U/L. In older males, it ranges from 10 to 48 U/L. The normal range in females is 6 to 29 U/L. Usually, elevated GGT levels signal a cholestatic liver process. Alternatively, elevated GGT levels occur within 24 hours of significant alcohol ingestion. When both alkaline phosphatase and GGT levels are elevated, the source of the alkaline phosphatase is most likely the liver. Note: GGT frequently rises above normal levels in response to the immune-stimulating effect of the Gerson Therapy.

Acid phosphatase

(not listed on example above)

Acid phosphatase, a group of phosphatase enzymes most active at a pH of about 5.0, appears primarily in the prostate gland and semen, and to a lesser extent, in the liver, spleen, red blood cells, bone marrow, and platelets.

Prostatic and erythrocytic enzymes are this group's two major isoenzymes; the prostatic isoenzyme is more specific for prostatic cancer. The more widespread the tumor, the more likely it is to produce high serum acid phosphatase levels. The acid phosphatase assay is usually restricted to adult males to detect prostatic cancer.

This test measures total acid phosphatase and the prostatic fraction in serum by radioimmunoassay or biochemical enzyme assay.

Purpose

To detect prostatic cancer and to monitor response to therapy for prostatic cancer; successful treatment decreases acid phosphatase levels.

Values

Serum values for total acid phosphatase range from 0 to 1.1 Bodansky units/ml; 1 to 4 King Armstrong units/ml; 0.13 to 0.63 Bessey-Lowery-Brock (BLB) units/ml; and 0 to 6 U/L in SI units, common to all these methods. Normal range of radioimmunoassay results is 0 to 4.0 ng/ml.

Implications of results

Generally, high prostatic acid phosphatase levels indicate a tumor that has spread beyond the prostatic capsule. If the tumor has metastasized to bone, high acid phosphatase levels are accompanied by high alkaline phosphatase levels, reflecting increased osteoblastic activity.

Misleading results may occur if alkaline phosphatase levels are high, because acid and alkaline phosphatase enzymes are very similar and differ mainly in the optimum pH ranges. Some alkaline phosphatase may react at a lower pH and thus be detected as acid phosphatase. Acid phosphatase levels rise moderately in prostatic infarction, Paget's disease (some patients), Gaucher's disease, and occasionally, in other conditions, such as multiple myeloma.

10. SGPT/ALT

(Alanine transaminase, serum; glutamic-pyruvic transaminase, serum)

Alanine aminotransferase (ALT), one of the two enzymes that catalyzes a reversible amino group transfer reaction in the Krebs cycle (citric acid or tricarboxylic acid cycle), is necessary for tissue energy production. Unlike aspartate aminotransferase, the other aminotransferase, ALT primarily appears in hepatocellular cytoplasm, with lesser amounts in the kidneys, heart, and skeletal muscles, and is a relatively specific indicator of acute hepatocellular damage. When such damage occurs, ALT is released from the cytoplasm into the bloodstream, often before jaundice appears, resulting in abnormally high serum levels that may not return to normal for days or weeks. This test measures serum ALT levels, using the spectrophotometric or the colorimetric method.

Purpose

• To help detect and evaluate treatment of acute hepatic disease - especially hepatitis, and cirrhosis without jaundice.

• To help distinguish between myocardial and hepatic tissue damage (used with aspartate aminotransferase [AST]).

• To assess hepatotoxicity of some drugs.

Values

ALT levels by a commonly used method range from 10 to 32 U/L; in women, from 9 to 24 U/L. The normal range for infants is twice that of adults.

Implications of results

Very high ALT levels: (up to 50 times normal) suggest viral or severe drug-induced hepatitis, or other hepatic disease with extensive necrosis. (AST levels are also elevated but usually to a lesser degree.)

Moderate-to-high levels: may indicate infectious mononucleosis, chronic hepatitis, intrahepatic cholestasis or cholecystitis, early or improving acute viral hepatitis, or severe hepatic congestion due to heart failure.

Slight-to-moderate elevations of ALT: (usually with higher increases in AST levels) may appear in any condition that produces acute hepatocellular injury - such as active cirrhosis, and drug- induced or alcoholic hepatitis.

Marginal elevations: occasionally occur in acute myocardial infarction, reflecting secondary hepatic congestion or the release of small amounts of ALT from myocardial tissue.

Interfering factors

Opiate analgesics (morphine, codeine, meperidine) may falsely elevate ALT levels by increasing intrabiliary pressure.

11. Alkaline phosphatase

This test measures serum levels of alkaline phosphatase, an enzyme that is most active at about pH 9.0. Alkaline phosphatase influences bone calcification and lipid and metabolite transport. Total serum levels reflect the combined activity of several alkaline phosphatase isoenzymes found in the liver, bones, kidneys, intestinal lining, and placenta. Bone and liver alkaline phosphatase are always present in adult serum, with liver alkaline phosphatase most prominent - except during the third trimester of pregnancy (when the placenta originates about half of all alkaline phosphatase). The intestinal variant of this enzyme can be a normal component (in less than 10% of normal patients; a genetically controlled characteristic found almost exclusively in the sera of blood groups B and 0); or it can be an abnormal finding associated with hepatic disease.

The alkaline phosphatase test is particularly sensitive to mild biliary obstruction and is a primary indicator of space-occupying hepatic lesions; additional liver function studies are usually required to identify hepatobiliary disorders. Its most specific clinical application is in the diagnosis of metabolic bone disease.

Purpose

• To detect and identify skeletal diseases, primarily characterized by marked osteoblastic activity.

• To detect local hepatic lesions causing biliary obstruction, such as tumor or abscess.

• To supplement information from other liver function studies and GI enzyme tests.

• To assess response to vitamin D in the treatment of deficiency-induced rickets.

Values

The normal range of serum alkaline phosphatase varies with the laboratory method used. Total alkaline phosphatase levels range from 30 to 120 U/L in adults; 40 to 200 U/L in children. Since alkaline phosphatase concentrations rise during active bone formation and growth, infants, children, and adolescents normally have high levels that may be three times as high as those of adults. Pregnancy also causes a physiologic rise in alkaline phosphatase levels.

Normal range is from 1.5 to 4 Bodansky units/dl; for the King-Armstrong method, normal adult values range from 4 to 13.5 King-Armstrong units/dl; 0.8 to 2.5 Bessey-Lowry units/dl; and 30 to 110 U/L by SMA 1260.

Implications of results

Significant alkaline phosphatase elevations are most likely to indicate skeletal disease, or extra or intrahepatic biliary obstruction causing cholestasis. Many acute hepatic diseases cause alkaline phosphatase elevations before any change in serum bilirubin levels. Moderate rise in alkaline phosphatase levels may reflect acute biliary obstruction from hepatocellular inflammation in active cirrhosis, mononucleosis, and viral hepatitis. Moderate increases are also seen in osteomalacia and deficiency-induced rickets.

Sharp elevations of alkaline phosphatase levels may result from complete biliary obstruction by malignant or infectious infiltrations or fibrosis. Such markedly high levels are most common in Paget's disease and, occasionally, in biliary obstruction, extensive bone metastases, or hyperparathyroidism. Metastatic bone tumors resulting from pancreatic cancer raise alkaline phosphatase levels without a concomitant rise in AST levels.

Isoenzyme fractionation and additional enzyme tests - serum gamma glutamyl transferase, acid phosphatase, 5'-nucleotidase, and leucine aminopeptidase - are sometimes performed when the cause of alkaline phosphatase elevations (skeletal or hepatic disease) is in doubt. Rarely, low serum alkaline phosphatase levels are associated with hypophosphatasia and protein or magnesium deficiency.

12(a). Cholesterol, total

This test, the quantitative analysis of serum cholesterol, measures the circulating levels of free cholesterol and cholesterol esters; it reflects the level of the two forms in which this biochemical compound appears in the body.

Cholesterol, a structural component in cell membranes and plasma lipoproteins, is both absorbed from the diet and synthesized in the liver and other body tissues. It contributes to the formation of adrenocorticoid steroids, bile salts, and androgens and estrogens.

A diet high in saturated fat raises cholesterol levels by stimulating absorption of lipids, including cholesterol, from the intestine; a diet low in saturated fat lowers them. Elevated total serum cholesterol levels are associated with an increased risk ofatherosclerotic cardiovascular disease, particularly coronary artery disease (CAD).

Purpose

- To assess the risk of CAD.
- To evaluate fat metabolism.
- To aid diagnosis of nephrotic syndrome, pancreatitis, hepatic disease, hypothyroidism, and hyperthyroidism.

Values

Total cholesterol concentrations vary with age and sex, and commonly range from 150 to 200 mg/dl.

Implications of results

The desirable blood cholesterol level is below 200 mg/dl. cholesterol levels of 200 to 240 mg/dl are considered borderline or at high risk for CAD, depending on other concurrent risk factors. Cholesterol levels that exceed 250 mg/dl indicate high risk of cardiovascular disease and require treatment.

Elevated serum cholesterol (hypercholesterolemia) may indicate incipient hepatitis, lipid disorders, bile duct blockage, nephrotic syndrome, obstructive jaundice, pancreatitis, and hypothyroidism.

Hypercholesterolemia caused by high dietary intake requires modification of eating habits and, possibly, medication to retard absorption of cholesterol.

Low serum cholesterol (hypocholesterolemia) is commonly associated with malnutrition, cellular necrosis of the liver, and hyperthyroidism. Abnormal cholesterol levels frequently necessitate further testing to pinpoint the disorder, depending on the type of abnormality and the presence of overt signs. Abnormal levels associated with cardiovascular diseases, for example, may necessitate lipoprotein phenotyping. ***Note:*** *Cholesterol levels often drop below normal levels in Gerson Therapy patients due to the extremely low fat nature of the diet, such results are not clinically* *significant in this context.*

Interfering factors

Cholesterol levels are lowered by cholestyramine, clofibrate, colestipol, cholchicine, dextrothyroxine, estrogen, dilantin, glucagon, heparin, kanamycin, haloperidol, neomycin, niacin, nitrates, para-aminosalicylic acid, and chlortetracycline. Levels are raised by adrenocorticotropic hormone, corticosteroids, androgens, bile salts, epinephrine, chlorpromazine, trifluoperazine, oral contraceptives, salicylates, thiouracils, and trimethadione. Androgens may have a variable effect on cholesterol levels. Failure to follow dietary restrictions may interfere with test results.

12(b). Lipoprotein-cholesterol fractionation

Cholesterol fractionation tests isolate and measure the cholesterol in serum - low-density lipoproteins (LDL) and high-density lipoproteins (HDL) - by ultracentrifugation or electrophoresis. The cholesterol in LDL and HDL fractions is significant, since the Framingham Heart Study has shown that cholesterol in HDL is inversely related to the incidence of coronary artery disease (CAD) - the higher the HDL level, the lower the incidence of CAD; conversely, the higher the LDL level, the higher the incidence of CAD.

Note: *A minimal amount of fat is essential in the diet and is included in the Gerson Therapy to provide an adequate supply of certain polyunsaturated fatty acids (the essential fatty acids) and of fat-soluble vitamins which cannot be synthesized in adequate amounts for optimal body function. As well as acting as a carrier of these essential compounds, dietary fat is necessary for their efficient absorption from the gastrointestinal tract.*

Purpose

- To assess the risk of CAD.

Values

Since normal cholesterol values vary according to age, sex, geographic region, and ethnic group, check the laboratory for normal values. An alternate method (measuring cholesterol and triglyceride levels, and separating out HDL by selective precipitation and using these values to calculate LDL) provides normal HDL-cholesterol levels that range from 29 to 77 mg/100 ml and normal LDL-cholesterol levels that range from 62 to 185 mg/100 ml.

Implications of results

High LDL levels increase the risk of CAD. Elevated HDL levels generally reflect a healthy state but can also indicate chronic hepatitis, early-stage primary biliary cirrhosis, or alcohol consumption. Rarely, a sharp rise (to as high as 100 mg/dl) in a second type of HDL [alpha(2)-HDL] may signal CAD. Although cholesterol fractionation provides valuable information about the risk of heart disease, other sources of such risk - diabetes mellitus, hypertension, cigarette smoking - are at least as important.

13. Triglycerides, serum

This test provides quantitative analysis of triglycerides - the main storage form of lipids - which constitute about 95% of fatty tissue. Although not in itself diagnostic, serum triglyceride analysis permits early identification of hyperlipemia (characteristic in nephrotic syndrome and other conditions) and the risk of coronary artery disease (CAD).

Triglycerides consist of one molecule of glycerol bonded to three molecules of fatty acids (usually some combination of stearic, oleic, and palmitic). Thus, the degradation of triglycerides is associated with several lipid aggregates, primarily chylomicrons, whose major function is transport of dietary triglycerides. When present in serum, chylomicrons produce a cloudiness that interferes with many laboratory tests.

Purpose

- To determine the risk of CAD.
- To screen for hyperlipemia.
- To identify disorders associated with altered triglyceride levels.

Values

Triglyceride values are age-related. Some controversy exists over the most appropriate normal ranges, but the following are fairly widely accepted:

Age	**Triglycerides**	
	mg/dl	mmol/L
0-29	10-140	0.1-1.55
30-39	10-150	0.1-1.65
40-49	10-160	0.1-1.75
50-59	10-190	0.1-2.10

Implications of results

Increased or decreased serum triglyceride levels merely suggest a clinical abnormality, and additional tests are required for definitive diagnosis. For example, measurement of cholesterol may also be necessary, since cholesterol and triglycerides vary independently.

High levels: of triglyceride and

cholesterol reflect an exaggerated risk ofatherosclerosis or CAD.

Mild-to-moderate: increase in serum triglyceride levels indicates biliary obstruction, diabetes, nephrotic syndrome, endocrinopathies, or excessive consumption of alcohol. Markedly increased levels without an identifiable cause reflect congenital hyperlipoproteinemia and necessitate lipoprotein phenotyping to confirm diagnosis.

Note: *Increased levels are sometimes seen in flare ups and reactions on Gerson Therapy and are of no negative clinical significance.*

Decreased serum levels are rare, occurring primarily in malnutrition or abetalipoproteinemia. In the latter, serum is virtually devoid of beta-lipoproteins and triglycerides, because the body lacks the capacity to transport preformed triglycerides from the epithelial cells of the intestinal mucosa or from the liver.

14,15,16,17. Protein electrophoresis, serum

This test measures serum albumin and globulins, the major blood proteins, in an electric field by separating the proteins according to their size, shape, and electric charge at pH 8.6. Because each protein fraction moves at a different rate, this movement separates the fractions into recognizable and measurable patterns.

Albumin, which comprises more than 50% of total serum protein, maintains oncotic pressure (preventing leakage of capillary plasma), and transports substances that are insoluble in water alone, such as bilirubin, fatty acids, hormones, and drugs. Four types of globulins exist - alpha(l), alpha(2), beta, and gamma. The first three types act primarily as carrier proteins that transport lipids, hormones, and metals through the blood. The fourth type, gamma globulin, is an important component in the body's immune system.

Electrophoresis is the most current method for measuring serum proteins. However, determinations of total protein and albumin-globulin (A-G) ratio are still commonly performed. When the relative percent of each component protein fraction is multiplied by the total protein concentration, the proportions can be converted into absolute values. Regardless of test method, however, a single protein fraction is rarely significant by itself. The usual clinical indication for this test is suspected hepatic disease or protein deficiency.

Purpose

• To aid diagnosis of hepatic disease, protein deficiency, blood dyscrasias, renal disorders, and gastrointestinal and neoplastic diseases.

Values –
Normal levels range as follows:

Total serum protein	6.6-7.9 g/dl
Albumin fraction	3.3-4.5 g/dl
Alpha(l)-globulin fraction	0.1-0.4 g/dl
Alpha(2)-globulin	0.5-1.0 g/dl
Beta globulin	0.7-1.2 g/dl
Gamma globulin	0.5-1.6 g/dl

Implications of results

The A-G ratio, the balance between total albumin and total globulin, is usually evaluated in relation to the total protein level. A low total protein and a reversed A-G ratio (decreased albumin and elevated globulins) suggest chronic liver disease. A normal total protein with a reversed A-G ratio suggests myeloproliferative disease (leukemia, Hodgkin's disease) or certain chronic infectious diseases (tuberculosis, chronic hepatitis).

18. Blood urea nitrogen (BUN)

This test measures the nitrogen fraction of urea, the chief end product of protein metabolism. Formed in the liver from ammonia and excreted by the kidneys, urea constitutes 40% to 50% of the blood's non-protein nitrogen. The blood urea nitrogen (BUN) level reflects protein intake and renal excretory capacity, but is a less reliable indicator of uremia than the serum creatinine level. Photometry is a commonly used test method.

Purpose

To evaluate renal function and aid diagnosis of renal disease and to aid assessment of hydration.

Values

BUN values normally range from 8 to 20 mg/dl.

Implications of results

Elevated BUN levels occur in renal disease, reduced renal blood flow (caused by dehydration, for example), urinary tract obstruction, and in increased protein catabolism (as in burns).

Depressed BUN levels occur in severe hepatic damage, malnutrition, and overhydration.

Note: Due to initial decreased dietary protein intake, the Gerson patient's normal value is slightly under that considered normal for the average person.

19. Creatinine, serum

A quantitative analysis of serum creatinine levels, this test provides a more sensitive measure of renal damage than blood urea nitrogen levels, because renal impairment is virtually the only cause of creatinine elevation. Creatinine is a nonprotein end product of creatine metabolism. Similar to creatine, creatinine appears in serum in amounts proportional to the body's muscle mass; unlike creatine, it is easily excreted by the kidneys, with minimal or no tubular reabsorption. Creatinine levels, therefore, are directly related to the glomerular filtration rate. Since creatinine levels normally remain constant, elevated levels usually indicate diminished renal function. Determination of serum creatinine is commonly based on the Jaffe reaction.

Purpose

- To assess renal glomerular filtration and to screen for renal damage.

Values

Creatinine concentrations in males normally range from 0.8 to 1.2 mg/dl; in females from 0.6 to 0.9 mg/dl.

Implications of results

Elevated serum creatinine levels generally indicate renal disease that has seriously damaged 50% or more of the nephrons. Elevated creatinine levels may also be associated with gigantism and acromegaly.

Interfering factors

- Ascorbic acid (Vit. C), barbiturates, and diuretics may raise serum creatinine levels.
- Sulfobromophthalein or phenolsulfonphthalein given within the previous 24 hours can elevate creatinine levels if the test is based on the Jaffe reaction.
- Patients with exceptionally large muscle masses, such as athletes, may have above average creatinine levels, even in the presence of normal renal function.

20. Uric Acid, serum

Used primarily to detect gout. this test measures serum levels of uric acid, the major end metabolite of purine. Large amounts of purines are present in nucleic acids and derive from dietary and endogenous sources. Uric acid clears the body by glomerular filtration and tubular secretion. However, uric acid is not very soluble at a pH of 7.4 or lower. Disorders of purine metabolism, rapid destruction of nucleic acids (such as gout), excessive cellular generation and destruction (such as leukemia), and conditions marked by impaired renal excretion (such as renal failure) characteristically raise serum uric acid levels.

Purpose

To confirm diagnosis of gout and to help detect kidney dysfunction.

Values

Uric acid concentrations in men normally range from 4.3 to 8mg/dl; in women, from 2.3 to 6 mg/dl.

Implications of results

Increased serum uric acid levels may indicate gout, although levels don't correlate with severity of disease or impaired renal function. Levels may also rise in congestive heart failure, glycogen storage disease (type I, von Gierke's disease), acute infectious diseases (such as infectious mononucleosis), hemolytic or sickle cell anemia, hemoglobinopathies, polycythemia, leukemia, lymphoma, metastatic malignancy, and psoriasis.

Depressed uric acid levels may indicate defective tubular absorption (as in Fanconi's syndrome and Wilson's disease) or acute hepatic atrophy.

Interfering factors

- Loop diuretics, ethambutol, vincristine, pyrazinamide, thiazides, and low doses of salicylates may raise uric acid levels. When uric acid is measured by the colorimetric method, false elevations may be caused by acetaminophen, ascorbic acid, levodopa, and phenacetin.
- Starvation, a high-purine diet, stress and alcohol abuse may raise uric acid levels.
- Aspirin in high doses, coumarin, clofibrate, cinchophen, adrenocorticotopic hormone, and phenothiazines may decrease uric acid levels.

21. Glucose, fasting blood sugar (FBS)

Commonly used to screen for disorders of glucose metabolism, mainly diabetes mellitus, the fasting plasma glucose test measures plasma glucose levels following a 12-to 14-hour fast.

In the fasting state, blood glucose levels decrease, stimulating release of the hormone glucagon. Glucagon then acts to raise plasma glucose by accelerating glycogenolysis, stimulating glyconeogenesis, and inhibiting glycogen synthesis. Normally, secretion of insulin checks this rise in glucose levels. In diabetes, however, absence or deficiency of insulin allows persistently high glucose levels.

Purpose

- To screen for diabetes mellitus and other disorders of glucose metabolism.
- To monitor drug or dietary therapy in patients with diabetes mellitus.
- To aid determination of insulin requirements in patients with uncontrolled diabetes mellitus and in those who require parenteral or enteral nutritional support.
- To aid evaluation of patients with known or suspected hypoglycemia.

Values

Normal range for fasting blood glucose varies according to the laboratory procedure. Generally, normal values after an 8 to 12 hour fast are as follows: fasting serum, 70-100 mg/dl; fasting whole blood, 60 to 100 mg/dl; nonfasting, 85 to 125 mg/dl in persons over age 50, and 70 to 115 mg/dl in persons under age 50.

Implications of results

Fasting blood glucose levels of 140 to 150 mg/dl or higher, obtained on two or more occasions may be considered diagnostic of diabetes mellitus if other possible causes of hyperglycemia have been ruled out. Nonfasting levels that exceed 200 mg/dl also suggest diabetes. Although increased fasting blood glucose levels most commonly indicate diabetes, such levels can also result from pancreatitis, hyperthyroidism, and pheochromocytoma. Hyperglycemia may also stem from chronic hepatic disease, brain trauma, chronic illness, or chronic malnutrition, and is typical in eclampsia, anoxia, and convulsive disorders.

Depressed glucose levels can result from hyperinsulinism (overdose of insulin is the most common cause), insulinoma, von Gierke's disease, functional or reactive hypoglycemia, hypothyroidism, adrenal insufficiency, congenital adrenal hyperplasia, hypopituitarism, islet cell carcinoma of the pancreas, hepatic necrosis, and glycogen storage disease.

22. Iron, serum, and total iron-binding capacity

Iron is essential to the formation and function of hemoglobin, as well as many other heme and non-heme compounds. After iron is absorbed by the intestine, it's distributed to various body compartments for synthesis, storage, and transport. Since iron appears in the plasma, bound to a glycoprotein called transferrin, it is easily sampled and measured. The sample is treated with buffer and color reagents.

Serum iron assay measures the amount of iron bound to transferrin; total iron-binding capacity (TIBC) measures the amount of iron that would appear in plasma if all the transferrin were saturated with iron. The percentage of saturation is obtained by dividing the serum iron result by the TIBC, which reveals the actual amount of saturated transferrin. Normally, transferrin is about 30% saturated.

Serum iron and TIBC are of greater diagnostic usefulness when performed with the serum ferritin assay; together these tests may not accurately reflect the state of other iron compartments, such as myoglobin iron and the labile iron pool. Bone marrow or liver biopsy, and iron absorption or excretion studies may yield more information.

Purpose

- To estimate total iron storage.
- To aid diagnosis of hemochromatosis.
- To help distinguish between iron deficiency anemia and anemia of chronic disease.
- To aid evaluation of nutritional status.

Values:

Normal serum iron and TIBC values are as follows:

Serum iron	TIBC mcg/dl	Saturation mcg/dl
Men:		
70-150	300-400	20% - 50%
Women:		
80-150	350-450	20% - 50%

Implications of results

In iron deficiency, serum iron levels drop and TIBC increases to decrease the saturation. In cases of chronic inflammation (such as in rheumatoid arthritis), serum iron may be low in the presence of adequate body stores, but TIBC may be unchanged or may drop to preserve normal saturation. Iron overload may not alter serum levels until relatively late, but in general, serum iron increases and TIBC remains the same to increase the saturation.

23. Erythrocyte count (Red blood cell count)

This test reports the number of red blood cells (RBCs) found in a microliter (cubic millimeter) of whole blood, and is included in the complete blood count.

Traditionally counted by hand with a hemacytometer, RBCs are now commonly counted with electronic devices, which provide faster, more accurate results. The RBC count itself provides no qualitative information regarding the size, shape, or concentration of hemoglobin within the corpuscles but may be used to calculate two erythrocyte indices: mean corpuscular volume (MCV) and mean corpuscular hemoglobin (MCH).

Purpose

To supply figures for computing the erythrocyte indices, which reveal RBC size and hemoglobin content.

To support other hematologic tests in diagnosis of anemia and polycythemia.

Values

Normal RBC values vary, depending on age, sex, sample, and geographic location. In adult males, red cell counts range from 4.5 to 6.2 million/microliter (4.5 to 6.2 x 1012/L) of venous blood; in adult females, 4.2 to 5.4 million/microliter (4.2 to 5.4 x 1012/L) of venous blood; in children, 4.6 to 4.8 million/microliter of venous blood. In full-term infants, values range from 4.4 to 5.8 million/microliter (4.4 to 5.8 x 1012/L) of capillary blood at birth; fall to 3 to 3.8 million/microliter (3.0 to 3.8 x 1012/L) at age 2 months; and increase slowly thereafter. Values are generally higher in persons living at high altitudes.

Implications of results

An elevated RBC count may indicate primary or secondary polycythemia, or dehydration; a depressed count may indicate anemia, fluid overload, or recent hemorrhage. Further tests, such as stained cell indices, and white cell studies, are needed to confirm diagnosis.

Note: *If total bedrest has been ordered, RBC counts may commonly drop considerably due to decreased oxygen requirements.*

24. Hemoglobin (Hgb), total

This test, usually performed as part of a complete blood count, measures the grams of hemoglobin found in a deciliter (100rnl) of whole blood. Hemoglobin concentration correlates closely with the red blood cell (RBC) count, and is affected by the hemoglobin-RBC ratio (mean corpuscular hemoglobin [MCH]) and free plasma hemoglobin. In the laboratory, hemoglobin is chemically converted to pigmented compounds and is measured by spectrophotometric or colorimetric technique.

Purpose

- To measure the severity of anemia or polycythemia and monitor response to therapy.
- To supply figures for calculating MCH and mean corpuscular hemoglobin concentration.

Values

Hemoglobin concentration varies, depending on the patient's age and sex, and on the type of blood sample drawn. Except for infants, values for age groups listed in Normal hemoglobin levels are based on venous blood samples.

Normal hemoglobin levels

Age	Hemoglobin level
Less than 7 days	17 to 22 g/dl
1 week	15 to 20 g/dl
1 month	11 to 15 g/dl
Children	11 to 13 g/dl
Adult males	14 to 18 g/dl
Elderly males	12.4 to 14.9 g/dl
Adult females	12 to 16 g/dl
Elderly females	11.7 to 13.8 g/dl

25. Hematocrit (Hct)

Hematocrit (Hct) measures the percentage by volume of packed red blood cells (RBCs) in a whole blood sample; for example, an Hct of 40% (0.40) means that a 100-ml sample contains 40 ml of packed RBCs. This packing is achieved by cetrifugation of anticoagulated whole blood in a capillary tube, so that red cells are tightly packed without hemolysis. Hct depends mainly on the number of RBCs, but is also influenced by the average size of the RBC. For example, conditions such as elevated concentrations of blood glucose and sodium, which cause swelling of erythrocytes may produce elevated hematocrits.

Test results may be used to calculate two erythrocyte indices: mean corpuscular volume (MCV) and mean corpuscular hemoglobin concentration (MCHC).

Purpose

- To aid diagnosis of abnormal states of hydration, polycythemia, and anemia.
- To aid in calculating red cell indices.
- To monitor fluid imbalance.
- To monitor blood loss and evaluate blood replacement.
- To conduct routine screening as part of the complete blood count.

Values

Hct values vary, depending on the patient's sex and age, type of sample, and the laboratory performing the test. Reference values range from 40% to 54% (0.40 to

0.54) for men, and 37% to 47% (0.37 to 0.47) for women.

Implications of results

Low Hct may indicate anemia or hemodilution; high Hct suggests polycythemia or hemoconcentration caused by blood loss.

Note: *Post-test care. If a hematoma develops at the venipuncture sites, applying ice, followed later by warm soaks, eases discomfort.*

26, 27, 28. Erythrocyte indices Red cell indices

Using the results of the red blood cell (RBC) count, hematocrit. and total hemoglobin tests, the red cell indices provide important information about the size, hemoglobin concentration, and hemoglobin weight of an average red cell. The indices include mean corpuscular volume (MCV), mean corpuscular hemoglobin (MCH), and mean corpuscular hemoglobin concentration (MCHC).

MCV, the ratio of hematocrit (packed cell volume) to the RBC count, expresses the average size of the erythrocytes and indicates whether they are undersized (microcytic), oversized (macrocytic), or normal (normocytic). MCH, the hemoglobin-RBC ratio, gives the weight of hemoglobin in an average red cell. MCHC, the ratio of hemoglobin weight to hematocrit, defines the concentration of hemoglobin in 100 ml of packed red cells. It helps distinguish normally colored (normochromic) red cells from paler (hypochromic) red cells.

Purpose

• To aid diagnosis and classification of anemia.

Values

The range of normal red cell indices is as follows:

MCV:

84 to 99 microliters^3 /red cell(fL/red cell)

MCH:

26 to 32 pg/red cell

MCHC:

30% to 36% (300 to 360 g/L)

Implications of results

The red cell indices aid in classification of anemias. Low MCV and MCHC indicate microcytic, hypochromic anemias caused by iron deficiency anemia, pyridoxine-responsive anemia, and thalassemia. A high MCV suggests macrocytic anemias caused by megaloblastic anemias, caused by folic acid or vitamin B-12 deficiency, inherited disorders of DNA synthesis, and reticulocytosis. Because MCV reflects average volume of many cells, a value within normal range can encompass RBCs of varying size, from microcytic to macrocytic.

Erythrocyte sedimentation rate (ESR) Sed rate

(Not listed on example above)

The erythrocyte sedimentation rate (ESR) measures the time required for erythrocytes in a whole blood sample to settle to the bottom of a vertical tube. As the red cells descend in the tube, they displace an equal volume of plasma upward, which retards the downward progress of other settling blood elements. Factors affecting ESR include red cell volume, surface area, density, aggregation, and surface charge. Plasma proteins (notably fibrinogen and globulin) encourage aggregation, increasing ESR.

The ESR is a sensitive but nonspecific test that is frequently the earliest indicator of disease when other chemical or physical signs are normal. It often rises significantly in widespread inflammatory disorders caused by infection or autoimmune mechanisms; such elevations may be prolonged in localized inflammation and malignancy.

Note: *ESR is also frequently raised during and after reactions and fevers induced by the Gerson Therapy.*

Purpose

• To monitor inflammatory or malignant disease.

• To aid detection and diagnosis of occult disease, such as tuberculosis, tissue necrosis, or connective tissue disease.

Values

Normal sedimentation rates range from 0 to 20 mm/hour; rates gradually increase with age.

Implications of results

The ESR rises in pregnancy, acute or chronic inflammation, tuberculosis, paraproteinemias (especially multiple myeloma and Waldenstrom's macroglobulinemia), rheumatic fever, rheumatoid arthritis, and some malignancies. Anemia also tends to raise ESR, since less upward displacement of plasma occurs to retard the relatively few sedimenting RBCs. Polycythemia, sickle cell anemia, hyperviscosity, or low plasma protein level tends to depress ESR.

29. Platelet count

Platelets, or thrombocytes, are the smallest formed elements in the blood. They are vital to the formation of the hemostatic plug in vascular injury, and promote coagulation by supplying phospholipids to the intrinsic thromboplastin pathway. Platelet count is one of the most important screening tests of platelet function. Accurate counts are vital for monitoring chemotherapy, radiation therapy, or severe thrombocytosis and thrombocytopenia. A platelet count that falls below 50,000 can cause spontaneous bleeding; when it drops below 5,000, fatal central nervous system bleeding or massive gastrointestinal hemorrhage is possible.

Properly prepared and stained peripheral blood films provide a reliable estimate of platelet number if the sample shows at least one platelet for every 10 to 20 red blood cells visible in an oil-immersion field. A more accurate visual method involves use of a hemacytometer counting chamber and a phase microscope. The most accurate measurement, however, employs the voltage pulse or electro-optical counting system. Nevertheless, results from such automated systems should always be checked against a visual estimate from a stained blood film.

Purpose

- To evaluate platelet production.
- To assess effects of chemotherapy or radiation therapy on platelet production.
- To aid diagnosis of thrombocytopenia and thrombocytosis.
- To confirm visual estimate of platelet number and morphology from a stained blood film.

Values

Normal platelet counts range from 130,000 to 370,000/mm^ [130 to 370 x 10"/L].

Implications of results

A decreased platelet count (thrombocytopenia) can result from aplastic or hypoplastic bone marrow; infiltrative bone marrow disease, such as carcinoma, leukemia, or disseminated infection; megakaryocytic hypoplasia; ineffective thrombopoiesis caused by folic acid or vitamin B-12 deficiency; pooling of platelets in an enlarged spleen; increased platelet destruction caused by drugs or immune disorders; disseminated intravascular coagulation; Bernard-Soulier syndrome; or mechanical injury to platelets.

An increased platelet count (thrombocytosis), can result from hemorrhage; infectious disorders; malignancies; iron deficiency anemia; recent surgery, pregnancy, or splenectomy; and inflammatory disorders, such as collagen vascular disease. In such cases, the platelet count returns to normal after the patient recovers from the primary disorder. However, the count remains elevated in primary thrombocytosis, myelofibrosis, with myeloid metaplasia, polycythemia vera, and chronic myelogenous leukemia.

When the platelet count is abnormal, diagnosis usually requires further studies, such as a complete blood count, bone marrow biopsy, direct antiglobulin test (direct Coombs' test), and serum protein electrophoresis.

Interfering factors

Medications that may decrease platelet count include acetazolamide, acetohexamide, antimony, antineoplastics, brompheniramine maleate, carbamazepine, chloramphenicol, ethacrynic acid, furosemide, gold salts, hydroxychloroquine, indomethacin, isoniazid, mephenytoin, mefenamic acid, methazolamide, methimazole, methyidopa, oral diazoxide, oxyphenbutazone, penicillamine, penicillin, phenylbutazone, phenytoin, pyrimethamine, quinidine sulfate, quinine, salicylates, streptomycin, sulfonamides, thiazide and thiazide-like diuretics, and tricyclic antidepressants. Heparin causes transient, reversible thrombocytopenia.

30. White blood cell (WBC) count Leukocyte count

Part of the complete blood count, the white blood cell (WBC) count reports the number of white cells found in a microliter (cubic millimeter) of whole blood by using a hemacytometer or an electronic device, such as the Coulter counter.

On any given day, WBC counts may vary by as much as 2,000. Such variation can be the result of strenuous exercise, stress, or digestion. The WBC count may rise or fall significantly in certain diseases, but is diagnostically useful only when interpreted in light of the white cell differential and of the patient's current clinical status.

Purpose

- To detect infection or inflammation.
- To determine the need for further tests, such as the WBC differential or bone marrow biopsy.
- To monitor response to chemotherapy or radiation therapy.

Leukocytes White blood corpuscles. There are two types: granulocytes (those possessing granules in their cytoplasm), and agranulocytes (those lacking granules). Granulocytes include juvenile neutrophils (3 to 5%), segmented neutrophils (54 to 62%), basophils (0 to 0.75%), and eosinophils (1 to 3%). Agranulocytes include lymphocytes, large and small (25 to 33%), and monocytes (3 to 7%).

Not all leukocytes are formed in the same place nor in the same manner. Granulocytes are formed in the bone marrow, arising from large cells called megakaryocytes. Lymphocytes are formed in the lymph nodes and probably in bone marrow. Monocytes are formed from the cells lining the capillaries in various organs, probably principally in the spleen and bone marrow.

Function: Leukocytes act as scavengers, helping to combat infection. They travel by ameboid movement and are able to penetrate tissue and then return to the bloodstream. The direction of movement is probably due to the stimuli from injured cells, called chemotaxis. When invading bacteria destroy them, the dead leukocytes collect in the form of pus, causing an abscess if a ready outlet is not available.

Leukocytes, especially the granular forms, are markedly phagocytic, i.e., have the power to ingest paniculate substances. Neutrophils ingest bacteria and small particles; other cells such as the monocytes and histiocytes in the tissues ingest larger particles. They are important in both defensive and reparative functions of the body. Basophils most probably function by delivering anticoagulants to facilitate blood clot absorption or to prevent blood coagulation. Eosinophils increase in number in certain conditions such as asthma and infestations of animal parasites. Lymphocytes are not phagocytic. B-cell lymphocytes produce antibodies and T-cell lymphocytes are important in producing cellular immunity.

A greatly diminished number of erythrocytes is found in the anemias, and a greatly increased number of leukocytes (leukocytosis) is usually indicative of bacterial infection. A leukocyte count is usually taken preoperatively if infection is suspected, such as in appendicitis. A count may also be taken following surgery to be sure than an occult wound infection has not developed.

Values

The WBC count ranges from 4.1 to 10.9 x 10". Implications of results

An elevated WBC count (leukocytosis) usually signals infection, such as an abscess, meningitis, appendicitis, or tonsillitis. A high count may also result from leukemia and tissue necrosis caused by burns, myocardial infarction, or gangrene.

A low WBC count (leukopenia) indicates bone marrow depression that may result from viral infections or from toxic reactions, such as those following treatment with antineoplastics, ingestion of mercury or other heavy metals, or exposure to benzene or arsenicals. Leukopenia characteristically accompanies influenza, typhoid fever, measles, infectious hepatitis, mononucleosis, and rubella.

31. White blood cell (WBC) differential

Because the white blood cell (WBC) differential evaluates the distribution and morphology of white cells, it provides more specific information about a patient's immune function than the WBC count. In this test, the laboratory classifies 100 or more white cells in a stained film of peripheral blood according to two major types of leukocytes - granulocytes (neutrophils, eosinophils, and basophils) and non-granulocytes (lymphoctyes and monocytes) - and determines the percentage of each type. The differential count is the relative number of each type of white cell in the blood. Multiplying the percentage value of each type by the total WBC count provides the absolute number of each type of white cell. Although little is known about the function of eosinophils in the blood, abnormally high levels of these cells are associated with various allergic diseases and reactions to parasites. In such cases, an eosinophil count is sometimes ordered as a follow-up to the white cell differential. This test is also appropriate if the differential WBC count shows a depressed eosinophil level.

Purpose

- To evaluate the body's capacity to resist and overcome infection.
- To detect and identify various types of leukemia.
- To determine the stage and severity of an infection.
- To detect allergic reactions.
- To assess the severity of allergic reactions (eosinophil count).
- To detect parasitic infections

Reference values: White blood cell differential

For Adults:
Cells
(Rel. Value – Absolute Value)
Neutrophils
(47.6 to 76.8% – 1950 to 8400 microliters)

Lymphocytes
(16.2 to 43% – 660 to 4,600 microliters)

Monocytes
(0.6 to 9.6% – 24 to 960 microliters)

Eosinophils
(0.3 to 7% – 12 to 760 microliters)

Basophils
(0.3 to 2% – 12 to 200 microliters)

For children (age 6 to 17):
Cells
(Relative Value)

Neutrophils
(boys: 38.5 to 71.5%, girls: 41.9 to 76.5%)

Lymphocytes
(boys: 19.4 to 51.4%, girls: 16.3 to 46.7%)

Monocytes
(boys: 1.1 to 11.6%, girls: 0.9 to 9.9%)

Eosinophils
(boys: 1 to 8.1%, girls: 0.8 to 8.3%)

Basophils
(boys: 0.25101.3%, girls: 0.3 to 1.4%)

Interpreting the differential
To make an accurate diagnosis, the examiner must consider both relative and absolute values of the differential. Considered alone, relative results may point to one disease, while masking the true pathology that would be revealed by considering the results of the white cell count. For example, consider a patient whose white blood cell count is 6,000/microliter, and whose differential shows 30% neutrophils and 70% lymphocytes. His relative lymphocyte count would seem to be quite high (lymphocytosis); but when this figure is multiplied by his white cell count - 6,000 x 70% = 4,200 lymphocytes/microliter - it is well within the normal range.

This patient's neutrophil count, however, is low (30%) and when this is multiplied by the white cell count - 6,000 x 30% = 1,800 neutrophils/microliter - the result is a low absolute number.

This low result indicates decreased neutrophil production, which may mean depressed bone marrow.

An increase in neutrophils (polys) is found in the following:
1. Infectious processes, systemic: septicemia, pneumonia, meningitis, gonorrhea, diphtheria, poliomyelitis, herpes zoster, acute rheumatic fever, chickenpox, scarlet fever, erysipelas, peritonitis, and tetanus.
2. Infections processes, localized: pyogenic abscess, furunculosis, tonsillitis, mastoiditis, otitis media, sinusitis, cholecystitis, pyelitis, pyelonephritis, salpingitis, appendicitis.
3. Metabolic disorders: acidosis, uremia, gout, and eclampsia.
4. Drugs and poisons: digitalis, epinephrine, foreign proteins, venoms, mercury, lead, carbon monoxide, potassium chlorate, camphor, coal tar products, pyridine, benzol compounds, turpentine.
5. Acute hemorrhage: particularly when the hemorrhage is into a body cavity, e.g., ruptured tubal pregnancy.
6. Diseases of the hemopoietic system: myelogenous leukemia, erythremia, erythroblastosis foetalis, incompatible transfusions, sudden hemolysis.
7. Miscellaneous conditions: coronary occlusion, rapidly growing carcinoma, for twelve to thirty-six hours after major operation, burns.
8. Physiological conditions: strenuous exercise, pregnancy, labor, during digestion, after hot bath, fear, pain, dehydration, extreme sunlight and high altitude.

A decrease in neutrophils is found in the following:
1. Bone marrow damage.
2. B^/Folic acid deficit.
3. Lupus erythematosus.
4. Splenomegaly.
5. Anaphylactic shock.
6. Typhoid and malaria.

Eosinophils are increased in:
1. Blood diseases: eosinophilic leukemia, myelogenous leukemia, polycythemia vera, slightly in pernicious anemia, and menses.
2. Parasitic diseases: trichinosis, schistosomiasis, infestation with some intestinal parasites, and in massive infestation with Taenia solium and amebiasis.
3. Skin diseases: psoriasis, dermatitis herpetiformis, erythema multiforme, urticaria and angioneurotic edema. Also radiation exposure/therapy.
4. Neoplasms: Some cases of malignant granuloma (Hodgkin's disease), ovarian and bone neoplasms, and neoplasms showing extensive necrosis.
5. Allergic diseases of the respiratory tract: bronchial asthma, hay fever, and pollinosis.
6. Poisons: phosphorus, copper sulfate, camphor, and pilocarpine.
7. Disease of unknown or doubtful etiology: Loeffler's syndrome,

chorea, scarlet fever.
8. Specific infections: Brucellosis, tuberculosis.

Basophils are increased:
1. Blood diseases: basophilic leukemia, myelogenous leukemia, polycythemia vera, chronic hemolytic anemia.
2. Miscellaneous: sometimes in Hodgkin's disease, chickenpox, small pox, following splenectomy, colitis and myxedema.
Basophils are decreased in hyperthyroidism and hyperadrenalism.
Lymphocytes are produced by the spleen, tonsils, lymph nodes and other lymphoid structures. They support the physiological immune/defense mechanism.

Lymphocytes are increased in the following conditions with an increased white cell count:
1. Lymphocytic leukemia, infectious mononucleosis, pertussis, tuberculosis, congenital syphilis, secondary syphilis, rickets, thyroxicosis, and malnutrition.

Lymphocytes are increased in the following conditions with a normal or decreased white cell count:
1. Pernicious anemia, familial splenic anemia (Gaucher's disease), typhoid fever, influenza, undulant fever (Brucellosis), infectious hepatitis, German measles, and mumps.

Lymphocytes are possibly decreased in:
1. Myelocytic leukemia (with increased myelocytes).
2. Lupus erythematosus.
3. Neutrophilic (poly) leukocytosis.
4. Radiation exposure (acute-early).
5. Severely depressed immune-system-lowered healing capabilities.

Monocytes are increased in the following conditions: Monocytic leukemia, brucellosis, typhus fever. Rocky Mountain spotted fever, Kala azar, cutaneous leishmaniasis, malaria, trypanosomiasis, sometimes in Hodgkin's disease, Niemann-Pick's disease, Hand-Schiller-Christian's disease, poisoning by tetrachlorethane. A decrease is of no significance.

Plasma Cells: Plasma cells are not found normally in the peripheral blood. They are round cells with deep blue cytoplasm and an eccentric nucleus containing deep-staining chromatin arranged like the spokes of a wheel. Plasma cells are found in the peripheral blood in the following conditions: Plasma cell leukemia, scarlet fever, and chickenpox. May be present in multiple myeloma and serum reactions.

Leukopenia: (Less than 4,800 WBCs). **Usually due to a decrease in neutrophils. Causes:**
1. Acute and chronic infections: typhoid, brucellosis, miliary tuberculosis, overwhelming pyogenic infections.
2. Measles, rubella, small pox up to about the fourth day, influenza after third or fourth day, infectious hepatitis, sand fly fever (passataci fever), sometimes in infectious mononucleosis.
3. Aplastic anemia, agranulocytosis, aleukemic leukemia, relapse of pernicious anemia, chronic hypochromic anemia, Banti's syndrome, familial splenic anemia (Gaucher's disease).
4. Systemic Leishmaniasis, malaria except during paroxysm.
5. Certain drugs and poisons: sulfonomides, barbiturates, amidopyrine, benzol, dinitrophenol, thiouracil compounds, tridione, pyribenzamine, arsenic, quinine, chloramycetin, thioglycolic acid, nitrogen mustards, and most cytotoxic chemotherapy drugs.
6. Radiation: x-rays, radium, and radiation from atomic disintegration.
7. Portal cirrhosis, anaphylactoid shock, rheumatoid arthritis, Felly's syndrome, cachexia, and debilitated states.

Urinalysis (UA), routine

Routine urinalysis is an important, commonly used screening test for urinary and systemic pathologies. Normal urine findings suggest the absence of major disease. Abnormal findings suggest disease and mandate further urine or blood tests to identify it. The elements of routine urinalysis include the evaluation of physical characteristics (color, odor, and opacity); the determination of specific gravity and pH; the detection and rough measurement of protein, glucose, and ketone bodies; and the examination of sediment for blood cells, casts and crystals.

Urinalysis methods include visual examination for appearance; reagent strip screening for pH, protein, glucose, and ketone bodies; refractometry for specific gravity; and microscopic inspection of centrifuged sediment for cells, casts, and crystals.

Purpose
To screen for renal or urinary tract disease and to help detect metabolic or systemic disease.

Normal Findings in routine urinalysis

Element	Finding

Macroscopic

color	straw
odor	slightly aromatic
appearance	clear
specific gravity	1.005 to 1.020
pH	4.5 to 8.0
protein	none
glucose	none
ketones	none
other sugars	none

Microscopic

red blood cells
0 to 3/high power field

white blood cells
0 to 4/ high power field

epithelial cells
few

casts
none, except occasional hyaline casts

crystals
present

yeast cells
none

parasites
none

Implications of results

Variations in urinalysis findings may result from diet, nonpathologic conditions, specimen collection time, and other factors.

The following benign variations are commonly nonpathologic:

Specific gravity: Urine becomes darker and its odor becomes stronger as the specific gravity increases. Specific gravity is highest in the first-voided morning specimen.

Urine pH: Greatly affected by diet and medications, urine pH influences the appearance of urine and the composition of crystals. An alkaline pH (above 7.0) - characteristic of a diet high in vegetables, citrus fruits, and dairy products but low in meat - causes turbidity and the formation of phosphate, carbonate, and amorphous crystals. An acid pH (below 7.0) - typical of a high-protein diet - produces turbidity and formation of oxalate, cystine, amorphous urate, and uric acid crystals.

Protein: Normally absent from the urine, protein can appear in urine in a benign condition known as orthostatic (postural) proteinuria. This condition is most common during the second decade of life, is intermittent, appears after prolonged standing, and disappears after recumbency. Transient benign proteinuria can also occur with fever, exposure to cold, emotional stress, or strenuous exercise.

Sugars: Also usually absent from the urine, sugars may appear under normal conditions. The most common sugar in urine is glucose. Transient, non-pathologic glycosuria may result from emotional stress or pregnancy and may follow ingestion of a high-carbohydrate meal. Other sugars - fructose, lactose, and pentose - rarely appear in urine under nonpathologic conditions. (Lactosuria, however, can occur during pregnancy and lactation).

Red cells: Hematuria may occasionally follow strenuous exercise.

The following abnormal findings generally suggest pathologic conditions:

Color: Changes in color can result from diet, drugs, and many metabolic inflammatory, or infectious diseases.

Note: *Beets cause pink or even light red urine, often mistaken for bleeding by new Gerson patients.*

Odor: In diabetes mellitus, starvation, and dehydration, a fruity odor accompanies formation of ketone bodies. In urinary tract infection, a fetid odor is common. Maple syrup urine disease and phenyiketonuria also cause distinctive odors. Note: Asparagus causes a strong fruity odor which is of no clinical significance.

Turbidity: Turbid urine may contain blood cells, bacteria, fat, or chyle, suggesting renal infection.

Specific gravity: Low specific gravity (less than 1.005) is characteristic of diabetes insipidus, nephrogenic diabetes insipidus, acute tubular necrosis, and pyelonephritis. Fixed specific gravity, in which values remain 1.010 regardless of fluid intake, occurs in chronic glomerulonephritis with severe renal damage. High specific gravity (greater than 1.020) occurs in nephrotic syndrome, dehydration, acute glomerulonephritis, congestive heart failure, liver failure, and shock.

pH: Alkaline urine pH may result from Fanconi's syndrome, urinary tract infection, and metabolic or respiratory alkalosis. Acid urine pH is associated with renal tuberculosis, pyrexia, phenyiketonuria and alkaptonuria, and all forms of acidosis. Note: The Gerson Therapy causes constant alkaline tides in high urinary pH.

Protein: Proteinuria suggests renal diseases, such as nephritis, nephrolithiasis, polycystic kidney disease, and renal failure. Proteinuria can also result from multiple myeloma.

Sugars: Glycosuria usually

indicates diabetes mellitus but may also result from pheochromocytoma. Gushing's syndrome, and increased intracranial pressure. Fructosuria, galactosuria, and pentosuria generally suggest rare hereditary metabolic disorders. However, an alimentary form of pentosuria and fructosuria may follow excessive ingestion of pentose or fructose, resulting in hepatic failure to metabolize the sugar. Because the renal tubules fail to reabsorb pentose or fructose, these sugars. spill over into the urine.

Ketones: Ketonuria occurs in diabetes mellitus when cellular energy needs exceed available cellular glucose. In the absence of glucose, cells metabolize fat, an alternate energy supply. Ketone bodies - the end products of incomplete fat metabolism - accumulate in plasma and are excreted in the urine. Ketonuria may also occur in starvation states and in conditions of acutely increased metabolic demand associated with decreased food intake, such as diarrhea or vomiting.

Cells: Hematuria indicates bleeding within the genitourinary tract and may result from infection, obstruction, inflammation, trauma, tumors, glomerulonephritis, renal hypertension,- lupus nephritis, renal tuberculosis, renal vein thrombosis, hydronephrosis, pyelonephritis, scurvy, malaria, parasitic infection of the bladder, subacute bacterial endocarditis, polyarteritis nodosa, and hemorrhagic disorders. Numerous white cells in urine usually imply urinary tract inflammation, especially cystitis or pyelonephritis. White cells and white cell casts in urine suggest renal infection. An excessive number of epithelial cells suggests renal tubular degeneration.

Casts: (plugs of gelled proteinaceous material [high-molecular-weight mucoprotein]): Casts form in the renal tubules and collecting ducts by agglutination of protein cells or cellular debris, and are flushed loose by urine flow. Excessive numbers of casts indicate renal disease. Hyaline casts are associated with renal parenchymal disease, inflammation, and trauma to the glomerular capillary membrane; epithelial cast, with renal tubular damage, nephrosis, eclampsia, amyloidosis, and heavy metal poisoning; coarse and fine granular cast, with acute or chronic renal failure, pyelonephritis, and chronic lead intoxication; fatty and waxy cast, with nephrotic syndrome, chronic renal disease, and diabetes mellitus; red blood cell cast, with renal parenchymal disease, renal infarction, subacute bacterial endocarditis, vascular disorders, sickle cell anemia, scurvy, blood dyscrasias, malignant hypertension, collagen disease, and acute inflammation; and white blood cell cast, with acute pyelonephritis and glomerulonephritis, nephrotic syndrome, pyogenic infection, and lupus nephritis.

Crystals: Some crystals normally appear in urine, but numerous calcium oxalate crystals suggest hypercalcemia. Cystine crystals (cystinuria) reflect an inborn error of metabolism.

Other components: Yeast cells and parasites in urinary sediment reflect genitourinary tract infection, as well as contamination of external genitalia. Yeast cells, which may be mistaken for red cells, can be identified by their ovoid shape, lack of color, variable size, and frequently, signs of budding. The most common parasite in sediment is Trichomonas vaginalis, a flagellated protozoan that commonly causes vaginitis, urethritis, and prostatovesiculitis.

Appendix II: Newsletter Excerpts from the *Gerson Healing Newsletter*

Nutritional Superiority of Organically Grown Foods

Experimental evidence for the nutritional superiority of foods grown with organic fertilization

(Excerpted from the Gerson Healing Newsletter, Vol. 5, No. 2, 1989)

by Gar Hildenbrand

People who grow and eat organic produce like to tell other people that organic fruits and vegetables not only taste better, but that they are "better for you". People who grow and eat commercial produce tend to think that this is a lot of hogwash.

I remember stopping at a nice looking stand in a farmers' market to ask, "Is any of your produce organic?"

The farmer squinted at me, stonefaced, as though I had spoken to him in Swedish. After a short and uncomfortable silence, he answered, "Of course it's organic. If it grows in the ground it's organic."

I asked, "Do you spray it for insects?"

"Of course I do," he answered with a tone of exasperation; "you won't find bugs on any of my stuff."

I was already walking away from his booth as his voice dropped to a disgruntled mutter. I had decided a long time ago that whenever I could avoid pesticide exposure I would. I chose to eat organically grown foods because I reasoned that they were likely to be safer, considering especially the inadequacy of testing in the U.S. and the ineptitude and carelessness of the least competent handlers of these dangerous chemicals.

But, imagine with me for a moment what it might be like if pesticides were no longer a problem. Envision, if you will, a world in which consumer preference has eroded the market for foods grown with toxics. Instead, integrated pest management and biological controls are being used.

In this new scenario, will we really need organically grown foods anymore? Are they so much better than chemically grown foods?

To learn more, we must return to an unsettled argument about the different effects of pure chemical fertilizers versus organic composts.[1-3] This controversy has brewed since the turn of the century.[4-7] Commercial farmers use growth stimulating nitrogen, phosphorus and potassium (NPK) in sometimes very large quantities; organic growers fertilize with only farmyard manure and compost from chemical-free sources."

For many years, the U.S. Department of Agriculture has maintained that there is no discernible difference between conventional and organic produce[9] while organic growers have maintained that theirs is better.[10-12]

Some results of our survey

We found that early experiments support the possibility that organic methods can and do produce foods nutritionally superior for some species of animals. But they are not conclusive regarding the human population. Animal feeding experiments conducted in the 1920's by McCarrison[20] and later supported by findings of McSheehy[14] are compelling evidence that there is something fundamentally different and better about plants grown with the benefit of organic composts. In all these experiments, animals fed organically fertilized foods outperformed those fed chemically fertilized foods.

It has been established as scientific fact that plants derive nutrients from the soil.[15-19] In 1929, Rowlands and Wilkinson wrote in the British Medical Journal that their findings confirmed those of McCarrison.[20] In their rat study, they compared the healthy growth of rats fed organically fertilized seed with the abnormal growth and disease of rats fed chemically fertilized seed. They used vitamin B replacement to correct the poor health of rats fed "artificial seed", and proposed that such seed may be lacking in vitamin B.

That micronutrients non-essential for plant growth are important in animal and human nutrition is accepted.[21] Whether these micronutrients must be supplied by agricultural products is debated by industry.[22]

Some argue that all necessary nutrients are supplied by conventionally grown foods which are held to be exactly equivalent to organically grown foods in nutritive value.[23-26]

Advocates of organic growing methods are united around the idea that organically grown foods are nutrition-ally superior to chemically grown foods.[1-7,13,14,20,27-29]

Major differences of opinion stem from the discovery that plants of superior size and appearance can be grown in widely differing soils with the addition of large quantities of growth stimulating nitrogen, phosphorus, and potassium (NPK) fertilizer. USDA hailed NPK as a great advance in farming because its remarkably increased yields promised to feed the world.[30]

But comparisons of organic and chemically grown foods require much more concrete validation than can be supplied by beliefs, convictions and opinions, no matter how passionate or assertive they may be.

Best experiments

To my knowledge, the only scientific experiments of adequate design and sufficient duration to address questions regarding the composition of organic vs. chemically fertilized foods in terms of nutrients are those of Doctor Werner Schuphan, Professor, Lecturer, and for years Director of Germany's Federal Institute for Research of Quality in Plant Production.

In 1974, after thirty-six years of research comparing the soils and plant products of organic compost fertilization with those of chemical fertilizers, Schuphan published findings and conclusions based on a 12-year comprehensive experiment. Conclusions regarding importance of his findings to human nutrition were based on Schuphan's prior labors in human infant feeding experimentation.

Schuphan was definite and emphatic that organically fertilized foods (Stable Manure or Biodynamic Compost) are nutritionally superior to foods grown conventionally with either Nitrogen + Phosphorus + Potassium (NPK) fertilizer, or even NPK-amended barnyard manure fertilization. In Qual.Plant - PI.Fds.hum.Nutr. XXIII,4:333-358, 1974, Schuphan wrote, "That the consumer would benefit by the higher biological value of products of (fertilization by) Stable Manure and Biodynamic Compost is beyond question, as confirmed by... data based on 12 years' chemical investigations."

It is puzzling to me that excellent writers in the field, like Dietrich Knorr[31] and Katherine Clancy[27] who have both cited Schuphan's 12-year experiment, did not comment on its significance which derives from the strength and chronological length of Schupan's study designs. Perhaps the answer lies in *Qual.* Plant's clubfooted English translation of results of the 12-year study. That translation (in an otherwise generally excellent journal), with its frequently jabberwocky syntax could certainly have proved daunting to even their fine intellects.

I found the going very rough, but after some fretting and frustration over identification of idioms and grammatic intent, meaning surfaced gradually in the murky translation. Schuphan's solid experimental design and intelligent classical methodology revealed themselves in simple clarity.

Strong study designs

Knorr has written intelligently regarding the collective shortcomings of the majority of efforts to compare plant products of different methods and materials of fertilization. He has pointed[31] to three weaknesses common to most studies comparing organic and conventional agricultural systems: 1) the insufficient duration of the studies (most are only one or two years), 2) the choice of pots or plots instead of comparing whole systems (separate farms), and 3) the use of fresh weight (which is quite variable) with emphasis on yield and food quality (organoleptic tests for taste and smell), instead of more accurate dry weights and essential nutrient assays.

While it is true that Schuphan chose to use plots, their great number, the study's long duration, and the use of two different soils minimized the types of bias and error usually found in "flower pot" studies. For example, Schuphan's comparisons of yield for spinach, grown on four different fertilizers over five harvests, incorporated data from 130 separately planted plots. Measurements of nutrient content for potatoes represent data collected from 104 separately planted plots. Absolutely none of

Schuphan's findings were taken from only one harvest.

Rather than fresh (wet) weight, Schuphan used dry weight to measure yield, and conducted nutrient assays, soil tests, humus evaluations, and, importantly, toxicology tests.

Allaway called in 1975[32] for strong study designs and replications with emphasis on the inherent deficiencies in some soils. Schuphan has created a study with many replications which utilized both rich soil and nutrient-poor sand.

Through his conscientious efforts to be scientifically thorough, Schupan has far exceeded any measures necessary to comply with guidelines implied by both Knorr and Allaway. I am convinced that Schuphan's design has anticipated any of the usual critical attacks.

Schuphan's Study

To start, 25 concrete framed plots were filled with sand and 25 with fen (lowland rich soil). Each plot had 10 square meters surface (107.64 square feet) and was filled to a depth of .9 meters (2.95 feet). The top layer of the sand plots was mixed with a small amount of fen to improve water holding at the surface. The plots were designated to receive one of the following types of fertilization: a) NPK, b) Stable Manure, c) Stable Manure +NPK, or d) Biodynamic Compost.

It is important to note the exceptionally large quantity of Biodynamic Compost applied, equivalent to 38.38 tons per acre, in contrast to 13.39 tons of Stable Manure.

Biodynamic Compost and directions for its application were supplied by Dr. Heinze of the Forschungsring für biologisch-dynamische Wirtschaftsweise (Research Circle for Methods of Biodynamic Application) in Darmstadt-Eschollboicken.

The Stable Manure itself was of "low quality" (low nitrogen) and varied little from year to year. No notes were supplied by Schuphan, regretfully, regarding the nature of the animals nor their feed, e.g.: fresh grasses, grains, silage, hay. In future studies, such information could be valuable in comparisons of various Stable Manuring materials and practices. Likewise not supplied was information regarding the specific genetic strains of seeds.

Statistical significance

To test for conformity of yield, potatoes were planted in eight plots, four sand and four fen, and fertilized with Stable Manure alone. The strong statistical significance of the uniform results in these potatoes can be held as evidence for the reproducibility of the Biodynamic crops which, unlike all the others, were grown in only two plots per harvest (one fen and one sand).

With the exception of the Biodynamic crops, all other fertilizers were tested by planting each crop (e.g.: potatoes) in four fen plots and four sand plots per fertilizer per harvest, and by growing each crop a number of times over the 12 year period. Eight crops were rotated: spinach, lettuce, savoy (cabbage), potatoes, celeriac (celery root), carrots, fodder beets, and sugar beets. Most rotations were successional, meaning two crops per year in one plot.

Herein lies the strength of Werner Schuphan's studies. He has built an experiment within which is designed a protocol for simultaneous production of multiple replications. Additionally, he has analyzed a representative set of replications for reproducibility and has shown high statistical significance. With the exception of the Biodynamic fertilizer (due perhaps to the sheer weight of fertilizer required), all other experiments have been carried out four times on each of two soils per harvest. In this way, each crop was grown in 26 plots per harvest. That, ladies and gentlemen, is an excellent example of the traditional methods of the Golden Age of German Science.

Where applicable, results were averaged according to four morphological types represented by spinach, savoy, potatoes, and carrots.

Yield

Unfortunately, yield is the contemporary farmer's first concern. We have made it so. If, instead, his first concern were the nutritional value of the produce, his practice would be considerably different. The structure of our economy has not made it desirable or possible for the farmer to put his emphasis on biological value.

Schuphan found that organic fertilization could in no way compete in terms of yields with NPK. He wrote, "These data reflect at the same time the tremendous role of fertilizer practice on yield, and the function of the soil as a significant environmental factor influencing yield."

Dr. Schuphan chose NPK-stimulated crop yields as the representative norm. However, if growers adopt "biological value" as their primary goal, such gigantic chemically pushed yields may become impossible. Never-the-less, using NPK fertilization as the standard (100%) for conventional yield, the bar graph in figure one shows that Stable Manure by itself produces only a 54% yield on fen and an even lower 44% yield on sand. By comparison, Biodynamic Composting scored yields of 80% on fen and 72% on sand. The combination of NPK and Stable Manure produced the highest result, 117% yield on fen and 104% on sand.

It is important to note that Schuphan reported that representatives of Biodynamic management plans suggest that yields will be low for five building years.

Different plants

Considerable differences in yield are seen in Schuphan's comparison of spinach (a rosette), savoy (a large terminal bud), potatoes (a stem tuber), and carrots (a storage root). Highest yields in succeeding crops (two crops in one plot in one season) were attained on fen in 1963 by early savoy and carrots, followed by spinach and celeriac in 1969. In single main crops, fodder beets in 1968 led all others.

As expected, in comparisons of four different crops grown by the four methods of fertilization, increased yields of all NPK treated crops are remarkable. In spinach and in savoy, NPK surplus yields ranged up to slightly more than 80% above the competing fertilizers. In carrots, NPK yields were up to 53% increased, and in potatoes up to 41%. There was one surprising exception to this general rule: potatoes grown on Biodynamically fertilized plots yielded up to 19% above those grown on NPK.

Effect on soil

Soil analyses provided some surprises. Schuphan wrote, "Our expectations after 12 year's experimental work - that humus contents of soil would correspond to humus supply by organic matter - was not realized in fen soil."

Humus is the organic portion of the soil, from decaying plant and animal matter. It is rich with microbes. Theoretically, according to Schuphan, humus is thought to provide abundant plant nutrients which are released by warmth and moisture, the same conditions that stimulate plant growth.

Schuphan observed and reported an apparent paradox: Fen soil in those plots which received the largest yearly quantities of organic inputs (Biodynamic Compost and Stable Manure) tested with the lowest levels of humus at the end of 12 years of consecutive fertilization.

The breakdown was as follows: Fen soil in plots treated with NPK + Stable Manure exhibited the highest humus content on analysis, some 70+ mg/lOOg soil. In second place for humus content, again surprisingly, was soil from

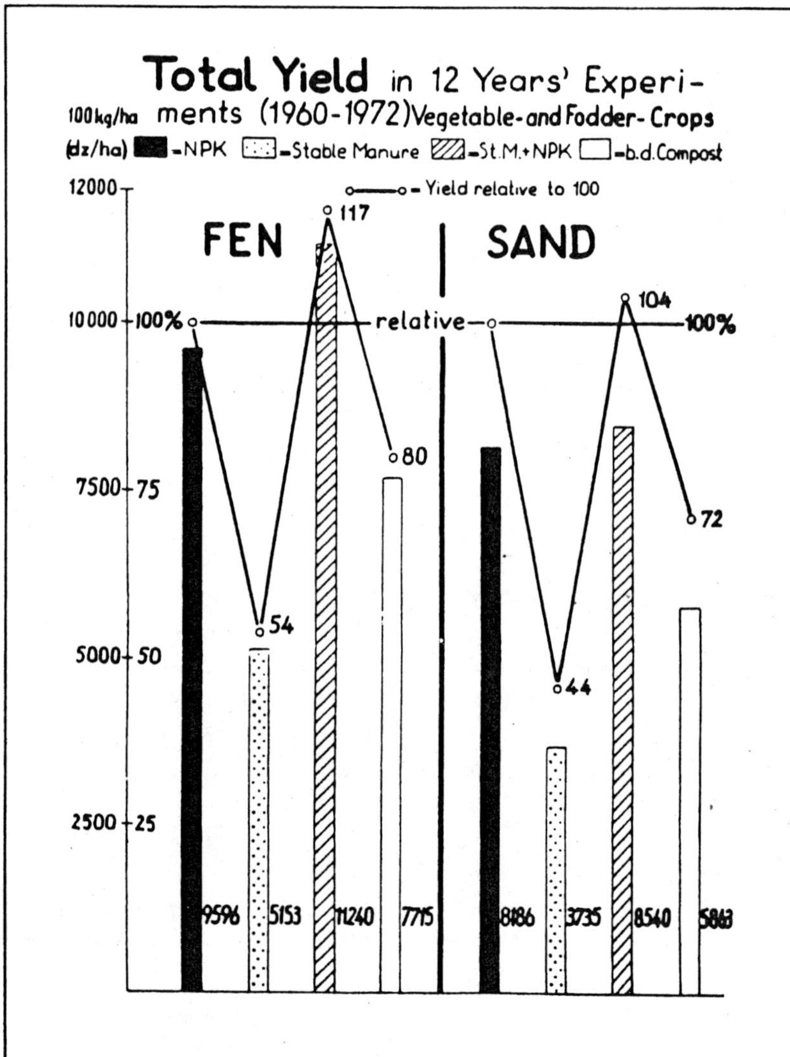

Figure 1

those plots treated with only NPK, at 67mg/100g soil. Third place went to plots treated with Stable Manure,

65mg/100g soil. Biodynamic Compost treated plots were tested at an astonishingly low 55 mg/lOOg soil, despite the addition of the equivalent of more than 38 tons per acre of Biodynamic Compost yearly for 12 years (compared to 13.39 tons/acre/year of Stable Manure).

Please look at the above paragraph again. Note that fen soil from NPK treated plots, which produced the highest crop yields, and which received absolutely no organic amendments, finished 12 years of consecutive, successional cropping with a higher content of humus than either those plots fertilized with Stable Manure or those treated with Biodynamic Compost. Why?

Schuphan did not attempt an answer. It is interesting to note that there was a very small buildup, especially with Biodynamic Compost, of humus in the sand-containing plots which received organic amendments. Again, Schuphan made the observation without discussion. Comparisons of humus and plant nutrients in fen and sand are not without difficulties.[33]

Schuphan conservatively avoided a discussion of mechanisms for the buildup of humus in NPK-treated soil. In addition, he reported extremely high contents of K_20, Fe, P_20s, Ca and Mn in fen soil plots treated for 12 years at with Biodynamic Compost. Rationalizing the latter, Schuphan suggested that low yields against high organic inputs might result in such mineral buildups.

More minerals in organics

Regardless of what was happening with the humus, the most important findings resulted from nutrient assays of crops.

In his own words, Schuphan reported: "Let us draw the most remarkable results to your attention. The most convincing facts are the much higher contents of minerals - with the exception of sodium - due to organic fertilizing. Potassium and iron show the greatest increases overall. Magnesium and calcium were also remarkably increased in savoy. Contents of sodium, with the exception of potatoes, are markedly decreased. "

In 1972[34], Schuphan pointed out that fruits and vegetables have a health-favoring" high potassium to low sodium and chloride ratio. This is directly opposed to animal products such as meat, milk, eggs, etc., which do not have a good ratio. Schuphan wrote, "It must be taken into account that according to our experimental results, attractivc cooking methods in which one cooks with plenty of water, throws away the cooking water, and seasons strongly with salt, cause an unfavorable partial displacement of minerals and significant loss of potassium. This points strongly toward the great value of pressed vegetable and fruit juices for dietetic purposes. "

More nutrients in organics

Just a few of the overall findings will suffice to show a trend. Compared with that grown on NPK-fertilized fen, spinach grown on organically fertilized fen soil contained from 64% (Biodynamic Compost) to 78% (Stable Manure) more ascorbic acid (Vitamin C).

In sand, spinach contained 30% (Biodynamic Compost) to 54% (Stable Manure) more ascorbic acid.

Savoy on organically fertilized fen contained 76% (Stable Manure) to 91% (Biodynamic Compost) more ascorbic acid. Savoy on sand tested at 64% (Biodynamic Compost) to 85% (Stable Manure) more ascorbic acid than that grown on NPK.

On fen soil, both Stable Manure and Biodynamic Compost increased the ascorbic acid content of lettuce by 59%. On sand, the increase was only 6% (Stable Manure) to 9% (Biodynamic Compost).

Against the trend toward higher nutrient contents, carotene-containing crops showed moderate decreases with organic fertilization, as much as almost 20% below the NPK norm. Schuphan noted that carotene is a "surplus product of plant metabolism, its synthesis being promoted by mineral fertilizing and favorable ecological conditions."

The need for more study, both of carotenes in biological (animal) systems, and of their intrinsic nature in plants, is obvious.

Proteins

Relative protein, a concern for those on limited diets, is increased in crops grown on organically fertilized fen soil. The increase in spinach is from 4% (Stable Manure) to 6% (Biodynamic Compost), in savoy from 33% (Stable Manure) to 40% (Biodynamic Compost), in lettuce from 15% (Biodynamic Compost) to 24% (Stable Manure), in celeriac 24% (Biodynamic Compost) to 37% (Stable Manure), and in carrots from 21% (Biodynamic Compost) to 25% (Stable Manure).

In potatoes, the increases were only slight, never as much as 10%.

In sand fertilized by organic inputs, the results were similar to the above, with a large difference showing only in carrots which were only barely higher than sand-NPK carrots.

Biological value of protein

The argument of organic vs. chemical fertilization hinges on two opposing issues: 1) maximum yield against 2) biological value.[34] Figuratively, biological value can be thought of as the sum of the actions of all components, both those that exhibit positive action like the vitamins, and those with negative action like the nitrates.[35] Schuphan's findings regarding amino acids and conjugated proteins in the above and the current studies throw much weight to the biological value side of the balance.

Heavy nitrogen fertilization results in a decrease in crops of the sulfur-containing amino acid methionine.[36,37] Methionine is essential in plant metabolism for the transfer of methyl (CH_3) from one compound to another. According to the above and earlier findings of Schuphan, diminished methionine content of crops due to heavy nitrogen fertilization results in decreased biological value of plant proteins.[38]

In the current experiments, both potatoes and spinach grown on organically fertilized fen and sand exhibited increases in methionine (expressed as a % of crude protein) from 11% to 47% above the NPK norms.

Schuphan observed a concurrent slight decrease in both glutamic acid and lysine in organically fertilized plants. In his opinion, enhancement of lysine content of crops, which increases with nitrogen fertilization, is not worth the loss of methionine and overall biological value of conjugated plant proteins. Lysine is touted by some nutritionists as playing a major role in the accelerated growth of young people of the Western World. It is richly supplied by animal foods of which there is plentiful supply. There is no need to devalue plant proteins in search of lysine stores for the public.

Schuphan wrote, "We may come to the conclusion that organic manuring un-equivocally favors sulfur-containing methionine, one of the most important amino acids. Breeders are very keen on genetically improving plant proteins by increasing their methionine contents. We have made it clear, however, that techniques of cultivation - more precisely, techniques of fertilization - may also help in this respect."

Less water weight In organics

Good looking, giant fruits and vegetables are considered desirable in the food industry. However, the measure of their food value is not their size and harvest weight, but rather their dry weight, which is a measure of their actual contents. Large, beautiful vegetables can be waterlogged and low in nutritional values. As one might suspect from the increased nutrient levels in organically fertilized crops, their dry weight is above that of their chemically fertilized counterparts.

Using chemically fertilized crops as the standard (100%), Schuphan demonstrated increases in dry matter in organically fertilized plants. In some crops treated with Stable Manure the gain in dry weight was as high as 69% above the NPK norm. Some crops treated with Biodynamic Compost ranged up to 96% beyond those fertilized with NPK.

Lower toxic nitrates

Schuphan earlier published[34] concerns regarding potential health hazards to infants of high Nitrate crops, especially over-fertilized spinach. In this study he wrote, "The most surprising result is the behavior of nitrate-N in spinach. Organic manuring both with Stable Manure and Biodynamic Compost results in extremely low contents of nitrate-N. No hazards to health whatsoever could be expected when such a "low-nitrate-spinach' was fed to infants."

Benefits In pest control

Nitrogen fertilized plants attract aphids more than is normal.[39] Observing that aphids require free amino acids from the stream of the vascular bundles of plants[40,41] Schuphan observed that organically grown plants are less susceptible to aphids for three reasons: 1) they have more collenchymatous thickening and subsequently more strength in cellular walls, 2) they have lower water content, and 3) they have lower contents of free amino acids.

Infant feeding studies

In a nine-year set of three separate infant feeding experiments[42-44] high contents of vitamins and minerals in crops were associated with health benefits to infants, including increases in daily weight gain, carotene in blood, vitamin C in blood, tolerance to teething, serum iron, and an improved red blood picture.

Schuphan points out that the nutritional constituents analyzed in the current studies are the same as those used to determine nutritional value in the infant feeding experiments which ran from 1936-1944. He asserts, "That is the reason why we claim validity for expressing our results in nutritional values."

Bottom line

On the whole, Schuphan's results support the argument that organic manuring produces foods which are nutritionally superior to those grown on chemical fertilizer. Let's look at some averages to help us to understand Schuphan's experimental evidence for the nutritional superiority of crops grown with the aid of either Stable Manure or Biodynamic Compost.

In comparison with NPK-fertilized crops which are assigned the relative norm of 100%, crops grown in both fen and sand with Stable Manure fertilizer or Biodynamic Compost fertilizer averaged higher in positive biological factors and lower in in negative factors (*Figures 2 and 3*).

Schuphan asserts that chemical fertilizers are used solely for a one-sided economic benefit to the food industry through remarkable increases in yield. In my opinion, this does not necessarily translate into gains for the farmer, whose commodities are therefore available often in such surplus that they are grossly devalued in a desperate effort to compete for buyers on the exchanges.[11]

Now that Schuphan has established a factual basis for the nutritional superiority of organically grown foods as they relate to human nutrition, let us look again at the experiments of McCarrison and McSheehy. Findings of this sort in animals, tied now to human nutrition through the labors of Schuphan, suggest the horrible reality that contemporary human nutrition constitutes a long term deficiency feeding experiment.

Standardization of organics industry practices must include generation and collection of the best scientific data regarding nutritional values in order to further the philosophical and practical knowledge and intent which gave birth to the industry. Industry credibility, which is vital, can be enhanced only by careful science.

It is important here to point out that Schuphan's results cannot be said to apply directly to all produce grown by various organic farming methods. It gives us some specific knowledge regarding several specific methods of organic fertilization and crop management. But what we are not told is far greater in scope than what we are told.

Factors having a positive biological Influence:

	NPK	Organic
Dry Matter	100%	123%
Relative Protein	100%	118%
Ascorbic Acid	100%	128%
Total Sugars	100%	119%
Methionine	100%	123%
(determined in potatoes and spinach only)		
Potassium	100%	118%
Calcium	100%	110%
Phosporus	100%	113%
Iron	100%	177%
(determined in spinach only)		

Figure 2

Factors having a negative biological Influence:

	NPK	Organic
Nitrates	100%	7%
(determined in spinach only in 1962,1969, and 1972)		
Free Amino Acids	100%	58%
Sodium	100%	88%

Figure 3

And we must therefore call for wide researches into nutritional qualities of foods grown by different methods of organic fertilization. Schuphan's twelve-year study with its basis in prior infant feeding experimentation should serve as a model for future researches. Other defined methods of organic growing should be put to similar tests.

Industry inertia is massive, and a way of doing business has been entrenched for many years which favors yield and cosmetics instead of biological value. But increasing numbers of consumers are more and more aware, vocal and active, sometimes militantly, against toxics and for nutritionally superior organically grown food.

There is a great, long journey ahead. But tomorrow holds hope if we will only pick up our bags and walk there.

References:

1. Rodal*, J.I.,(edito0, 'The Doctors' Attitude Toward Fertilizers' in Organic Gardening fJ-bra«yNo.1, Organic Gardening. 1847, Rodale Press, Emmaus, PA.

2. Howard, Sir Albert, 'An Agricultural Testament', 1940, Oxford University Press.

3. Vogtmann, H„ 'Effects of Agricultural Practices on Soil and Plant Quality'. ifoam BuH. 24:1-6,1978.

4. Howard, Sir Albert, 'The Soil and Health' Schocken Books, N.Y.

5. Grigga, B„ 'The Food Factor', 1986, Viking Penguin

Ltd., Hannondsworth, Middlesex, England.

6. McCarrlcon, Sir Robert, 'Nutrition and National Health'. 1936. Faber and Paber Ltd., 24 Russell Square, London. UK.

7. Balfou, Lady Eve, 'The Living Soil', 1943, Faber and Faber Ltd., 24 Russell Squa're, London. UK.

8. OFPANA (Organic Foods Production Assn. of North America), 'Guidelines for the Organic Foods Industry'. 1986. OFPANA. Box 31, Betehertown MA 01007, pg. 5.

9. USDA (U.S. Dept. Agriculture). 'Report and Recommendations on Organic Farming', July 1980, U.S. Gov't. Printing Office, pgs. §4-65.

10. Hardlng,T., "Opportunities in ag', AERO Sun Times, Spring 1987.

11. Harding, T,, "Organic Foods Production Association of North America', Complementary Mod., Sept./Oct. 1986, pp. 48-50; and 'OFPANA Seeks Uniformity, Commonality, Verification of Organic Foods', Whole Foods, Sept. 1986, pgs. 17-20.

12. Food Marketing Inatituto, 'Consumer attitudes and the Supermarker, 1987.

13. McCarrlson, Col. Robert 'The effects of manurial conditions on the nutritive and vitamin values of millet and wheat', Indian J.Med.Pes. 14:351-378.1927.

14. McSheehy.T.W., 'Nutritive value of wheat grown under organic and chemical systems offarming', Dual. Plant. -Pl.ds. Hum. Nutr. 27(2):113-123,1977.

15. Lilienthal, D., 'Nutrition and Soil Conservation', J.Am.Diet.Assn. 14:424-430, June-July, 1938.

16. Aucter, E.C,, USDA Chief of the Bureau of Plant Industry, 'The Interrelation of Soils and Plant, Animal and Human Nutrition', Scw1ce89(2315):421-427. May 12,1939.

17. Sherwood, F.W., el al, 'Effect of Fertilization on the Nitrogen, Calcium, and Phosphorus Contents of Pasture Herbage', Am.Soc.Agron.J.39{W):W,Oct. 1947.

18. Commonwealth Agricultural Bureau, 'Human and Animal Health in Relation to Soil Factors' (205 annotated references), 1977, Slough, UK.

19. Beeson, K.C., "The Effect of Fertilizers on the Nutritional Quality of Crops', Michigan State University, Centennial Symposium, pg. 45,1955.

20. Rowland*, M.J. and Wilkinson, B,, "The Vitamin B Content of Grass Seeds in Relationship to Manures', Biochem.J. 24:199-204,1930.

21. Bear, Firman E,, in 'Earth: The Stuff of Life', 1962, U. of Oklahoma Press, pp. 164-165.

22. Hopkins, H.T. I al, "Soil Factors and Food Composition", Amer. M. of Clinical Nutr. Vol. 18:390-395, May 1966.

23. Leverton, R,, "Organic, Inorganic: What They Mean", in 1974Yearbook of Agriculture. pp. 70-73, published by USDA, U.S. Gov't Printing Office.

24. Institute of Food Technologists 'Scientific Status Summary', Food Tecnnology 23. 71-74, 1974 (in Knorr, see ref. 31).

25. Packard, V.S., 'Natural? Organic? What Do They Really Mean?', Prof.Nut. 10(3): 1-3,1978.

26. Jukes, "The Organic Food Myth', JAMA. 230:276-277,1974.

27. Clancy, K.L., 'The role of sustainable agriculture in improving the safety and quality of the food supply, Am.J.Alt-Ag.. 1(1):11-16, Winter 1986.

28. USDA, 'Report and Recommendations on Organic Farming', pg. 11, July, 1980.

29. Svec, L.V. et al, 'Chemical Evaluation of Vegetables Grown with Conventional or Organic Soil Amendments', Commun. in Soil Science and PlantAnalysis. 7(2):213-228,1976.

30. USDA, "Yearbook', 1938: "Soils and Men" and 1939: "Food and Life'.

31. Knorr, D. and Vogtmann, H. "Quantity and Quality Determination of Ecologically Grown Foods' in "Sustainable Fooo Systems', 1983, AVI Publishing Co., Westport, Conn., pgs. 352- 381.

32. Allaway, W.H., 'The Effect of Soils and Fertilizers on Human and Animal Nutrition', USOA-ARSAg.Inf.Bull. No. 378, Wash.D.C.

33. Vetter, H. and Frdchtenicht, K., "Abstutung der Nahrstoff- Grenzwerte mit steigendem Humusgehalt', Landw.Forsch. 26:1-9,1973.

34. Schuphan, W., "Effects of the Application of Inorganic and Organic Manures on the Market Quality and on tne Biological Value of Agricultural Products', Oual.Plant.Mater.Veg. 21(4):381-398,1972.

35. Schuphan, W., 'Zur Qualitat der Nahrungspflanzen', BLV-Verlagsges., 1961, MOnchen, Bonn, Wien.

36. Oser, B.L., "Methods for integrating essential amino acid content in the nutritionaF evaluation of protein', J.Amer.Dietet.Assn. 27:396-402,1951.

37. Schuphan, W., "Methioningehalt und Eiweissqualitat von Biattpflanzen in Abhangigkeit von der StickstoffdOngung', Qual.Piant.Mater.Veg. 8:261-283, f961.

38. Schuphan, W., 'Der Einfluss einer steigenden N-OOngung auf den Gehalt an essentiellen Aminosauren und auf die Biologische Eiweisswertigkeit von Kartoffein (EAS-Index nach B.L. Oser)", i. Pflanzenem., DOng., Bodenkde. 86(131):1-14,1959.

39. Schuphan, W., "Problematik dOngungs-bedingter Httchstertrage aus phytochemischer und emahrungsphysiologischer Sichf, Qual.Piant.Mater.Veg. 25:35-64,1970.

40. Schaller, G., 'AminosAuren im Speichel und Honigtau der grtinen ApfelblaMaus Aphis pomi deg', Homoptera.Ent.exp.A appl. 4:73-85,1961.

41. Markkula, M. and Laurema, S., "The effect of amino acids, vitamins, and trace elements on the development of acyrthosiphon pisum Harris (Horn., Aphidiae)', Annales Agriculturaebenniae 0:77-80,1967.

42. Dost, F.H. and Schuphan, W., 'Ober Emahrungsversuche mit verschieden gedOngten GemOsen III', Die Emahrung 9:1-27,1944.

43. Schuphan, W,, Dost, F.H. and Schotola, H., 'Eine kritische Stellungnahme von Agrikulturchemie und Meaizin zur Frage der alTeinigen StallmistdOngung bei GemOse, Toil A undleil B', Die Ernihrung +5:29-37; 37-42,1940.

44. Wendt, H. et al, "Ober Emahrungsver-suche mit verschieden gedOngten GemOsen', Die Emahrung 3:53-69,1938.

Eat Only Organic

By Gar Hildenbrand and Christeene Lindsay

(Excerpted from the Gerson Healing Newsletter, Vol. 5, No. 1, 1989)

Readers of this newsletter have repeatedly and urgently expressed a desire to know what they themselves might do to improve their health and to prevent disease. In this day of miracle medicines and potent patented pills, what do the authoritative leaders, the frontier guides, of the Gerson Institute recommend? Is there some new supplement, some special herb, some .newly refined co-nutritive factor which might be the missing link?

Yes. We can make some recommendations:

Please eat an unsalted, very low-fat diet of "organically grown" fruits, vegetables and whole grains. Supply eight ounces daily of dense nonfat dairy protein (dry curd) or its equivalent in quite moderate amounts of animal products, mostly poultry and fish.

75% of the diet should be comprised of fruits and vegetables altered as little as possible, much of it raw and freshly prepared.

Please intelligently avoid all additives, including emulsifiers, preservatives, colorings, and flavorings even when these are labeled "natural" (an intentionally deceptive term).

When you cook, please use no fats (oil, lard, vegetable shortening, butter) and no cooking water. Use tightly covered bakeware at temperatures below the boiling point of water, allowing considerable additional cooking time. Do not overcook. It is not possible to fry at such low temperatures and without fat (oil).

Please allow no more than 25% of your diet to consist of meats, nuts, eggs, fish, cakes, cookies, candies, breads and other baked goods, and only if you enjoy excellent health. While we do not prohibit the use of red meats, they should be taken infrequently and then in moderation. Be aware that nuts and seeds of all types are sources of mostly fat. They should not be regarded as protein foods. While these are not prohibited foods, they are not part of the primary recommended diet, but rather an allowable addition. The moment your health declines, whether this involves infection, trauma (injury), poisoning, emotional/mental stress, or chronic disease, discontinue most of these marginal foods.

Time and time again

Why, in a world so modern, do we repeat these well worn recommendations? After all, on the strength of clinical observations, these same recommendations were already the accepted dietary wisdom of the Golden Age of German Medicine before WWII, when fruits, vegetables and dairy were called the "protective foods". In the U.S., these guidelines were brought forth in July of 1945, this time as prophylaxis against heart disease and cancer, before the U.S. Senate by the great German-American tuberculosis specialist, Dr. Max Gerson, pioneer of sodium restriction, potassium supplementation, protein-calorie restriction, and dietotherapy based on the protective foods.

Modern epidemiological observations have now confirmed the early 20th century clinical observations of the protective effect of fruits, vegetables, whole grains and dairy. Diets supplying predominantly these foods are inversely correlated to (they protect against) the incidence of our two great modern epidemics: cardiovascular disease and cancer.

The U.S. Senate's McGovern Committee reiterated them in 1977 as U.S. National Dietary Goals. The National Academy of Sciences' (NAS) National Research Council's (NRC) Committee on Diet, Nutrition and Cancer made the same recommendations in their interim dietary guidelines of 1982. The American Cancer Society (ACS) followed suit in 1983, and shortly thereafter the National Cancer Institute (NCI). Subsequently we have seen dozens of books based on these recommendations written by oncologists, cardiologists, physiologists, dietitians, nutritionists, journalists, reporters, and popular authors promising long healthy life without heart disease and cancer.

There is, of course, a direct correlation between food and health. It is nutrition which sustains us, and it is our food which nourishes us or destroys us.

What is nutrition? A good definition is found in *Taber's Cyclopedic Medical Dictionary*: "the sum total of the processes involved in the taking in and utilization of food substances by which growth, repair and maintenance of activities in the body as a whole or in any of its parts are accomplished. Nutrition includes ingestion, digestion, absorption, and metabolism".

Nutrition is responsible for repair not only in the rebuilding of damaged tissues, but also in the correction of disease through cell-mediated and humoral immunities. Nutrition is also responsible for maintenance of normal cellular integrity and tissue function, an important aspect of which may be characterized as resistance to disease.

All genuine authorities are now agreed on the relationship of diet, nutrition and health/disease. All informed laymen know it. Only a few sociopathic madmen and industrially sponsored prostitutes-masquerading-as-scientists continue to deny .it.

Then why do we repeat these recommendations? Because they are still not a matter of personal practice for the majority of the population. Although many possess an intellectual understanding of these guidelines, mysterious compulsions often act to override our intellects, leading us to consume exactly the wrong foods. This behavior can be observed even, and perhaps most clearly, in the most conscientious of us by auto-experimentation. Or it can be seen by paying close attention to coworkers, friends and family.

People fully knowledgeable of the negative health consequences of chronic food abuse, people who might lecture us regarding the evils of inappropriate diets, will give voice to their intentions to eat a diet fit for the human species and, in the next breath, will order a junk food pizza for dinner and invite their friends to join them. For many putatively healthy and sane adults, junk food consumption is the dominant dietary pattern when graphed over time.

Even if the relative quality of foods consumed is high, if the ratio of protective foods to the rest of the diet is insufficient, deleterious effects will result. Of course, many continually consume far too much high quality, hormone-free, organically fed meat, eggs, cheeses, fats, etc., in spite of knowing full well the high price which must eventually be paid to the piper.

We know of no satisfactory psychological theories or physiological explanations for the failure of our increasingly well-informed intelligent adult population to confront and correct its known suicidal dietary patterns.

But you can be different. You can become nutritionally streetwise and eat toward survival. You can stop worrying about vitamin and mineral pills as well as heart disease and cancer. You can also stop nervously reading labels for Recommended Dietary Allowances (RDAs), which as we'll explain later were never intended to be used by the individual seeking to improve his daily nutrition. All you really have to do is eat according to the original Gerson dietary guidelines which were part of the Congressional Record more than three decades before the printing of "Dietary Goals for the U.S.", and nearly four decades before the adoption of the same guidelines by NCI and ACS.

But there's a catch.
You must eat only "organic"

Not all fruits and vegetables are equally valuable. Methods of growing have an effect on the nutritive quality of foods. This effect, which is probably vastly beyond contemporary estimates, is currently immeasurable with the exception of a narrow group of markers known as nutrients and reflected commonly in the RDA tables.

Warning: Do not expect to find "organically grown" foods in all grocery stores. Purchase only those foods with certification labels clearly stating "organic". Foods grown by inappropriate technologies may actually be directly harmful to your health due to residues and/or metabolites of insecticides, fungicides, herbicides, rodenticides, and growth regulators. Such agricultural inputs frequently result in changes of the chemical composition and, presumably, in the steric (atomic spatial) relationships of molecules within the plants themselves. Thus, a commercially grown fruit which is apparently a beautiful apple may, in fact, be something quite different. Do you remember the story of Snow White?

In this issue, we will provide you with basic information about organic foods, what they are and how they are better than chemically grown foods. We'll look at who is growing them, who is selling them, and we'll provide you with information that will help you locate them. We'll also explain how you, personally, can help us to improve the safety and nutritional quality of the nation's food supply.

Quad me nutruit me destruit

That which nourishes me also destroys me. Man's food is his poison. Never before in history has this been so inescapably correct, for now as never before, we have plenty to eat and it is produced with plenty of poison.

What do we know of nutrition? Nutrients are molecular components of foods. They are observable and measurable and serve as markers for the evaluation of whole foods. They are correlated to normal plant growth and to health in humans. Some of them have been shown to prevent specific "deficiency" diseases such as pellagra, kwashiorkor, beriberi, rickets, night blindness, anemia and scurvy.

But there is more to nutrition than the known nutrients.

The erroneous impression has been created that a science exists in which the multiple processes of nutrition are understood. Nutrition has been observed. Some of the key nutrients - some of them - have been identified and extensively studied. These are proteins, fats, carbohydrates, vitamins and minerals. Components of the living organism of man have been similarly studied. However, our studies have just begun.

The marriage of the medical sciences (based in wet chemistry) with particle physics (quantum mechanics) has left us freshly astonished at the foot of a great mountain, facing our basic lack of understanding of the workings of living organisms.

At the subatomic level, man and plant are only vaguely comprehended by us. The actual dynamics of the myriad interactions between these are enigmatic, shrouded and invisible. Oftentimes, we don't even know what we are looking at. Are we perhaps studying the effects of our attempts to observe?

All that we know is gross, mechanical and simplistic. Honesty forces us to admit that every physiological system we have studied and mapped must now be incorporated into a new understanding, into a metasystem, in which, for example, a pancreas is composed of interacting electron shells and a gallbladder's functions relate to its neutrons and mu-mesons and charming quarks.

Suddenly, we find ourselves in an expansive realm where we have to admit that Benveniste's homeopathic experimental antigen reactions produced with water dilutions at the 120th power need not be explicable for them to be real. (If you are unfamiliar with these experiments, please read "The haunting of Nature" below.) Is it so inconceivable that water might "remember", might carry a "homeopathic ghost", when all matter is thought to be made up of energy/mass "wavicles" called quanta which themselves exist only intermittently?

Add to our overwhelming ignorance of the actual workings of life the horrifying knowledge that we are continually manufacturing chemical death messages and spraying them onto our agricultural commodities. These death messages are present at high dilutions in the living water of fruits and vegetables sold to the public. No one knows what they are doing. No one.

The authors have spent considerable time investigating pesticide safety testing, tolerances, residue-monitoring, and protection of the public. We've come to hold some very strong opinions simply stated as follows:

Our foods are poisoned. Fresh fruits, vegetables, and grains grown in this country are saturated with poisons which are capable of producing both acute and long-term negative health effects. Complicating this is the importation of 26% of all fruits and vegetables consumed annually in the United States, foods which are even more thoroughly contaminated than those produced domestically.

Our government Is not protecting us. The supermarket shelves, restaurants, and dinner tables of the United States of America are daily poisoned by an enemy from within. The system used by the Environmental Protection Agency (EPA) to establish so-called "safe" levels of residues is methodologically unsound. Serious flaws in logic stemming from factual errors and incorrect assumptions have propelled EPA to act exactly contrary to its Congressional charter. EPA has failed to remove almost all known disease causing agricultural chemotherapy products from the market and has, this year, unbelievably deregulated previously controlled hazardous agricultural chemicals. What is worse, we have no protection from the responsible regulatory body, the Food and Drug Administration (FDA), an agency as dysfunctional and inept as a chronic alcoholic and as dangerous as a drunken driver.

Pesticides are damaging this nation's health. America's economy is being relentlessly eroded by lost worker productivity and monumentally disproportionate health care costs. Added to this is the tragic economic collapse of the traditional American family farming system, which suffers from both the unanswerable financial challenges and the toxic side effects of long term aggressive agricultural chemotherapy.

Just as our finest physicians are powerless to either diagnose or treat the uncharted, often unrecognized maladies resulting from chronic exposure to agricultural chemicals, our top agricultural scientists are impotent in the face of multi-pesticide-resistant predators, insects and plant diseases.

Far from providing a permanent answer to the need for worldwide supplies of agricultural commodities, conventional farm chemotherapy threatens to kill the patient through disruption of living soil ecosystems, and may very well send the rest of us to the gallows, our bellies full with "the prisoners last meal".

In the context of this newsletter we will provide powerful statements from this nation's elected officials and other leading authoritative critics of conventional farm chemotherapy. You will be privy to a battle being fought in Washington which has been unreported to the American people in one of the most curious media blackouts we at the Gerson Institute have ever seen.

This nation's media are a mix of responsible genius, competence, incompetence, idiocy, and unethical behavior. It is a difficult job to sort out the truth from the propaganda, as often the journalists themselves are relatively innocent and manipulated by apparent authorities.

This is an era in which Commissioner Frank Young of the FDA entered office in 1984 touting the "anti-quack" platform, a "safe" platform to be sure, but one which has no constructive essence. Anti-quackery is a bandwagon easy to hop. Only last year, the Los Angeles Times ran journalist John Hurst's insensitive and stupidly inaccurate "quack trashing" articles, attacking Charlotte Gerson and Dr. Max Gerson. The LA Times refused to print our letters in response to Hurst who was inspired by writers for the National Council Against Health Fraud, a self-promoting group of "quackbashing" grandstanders who seek to make themselves taller by cutting off the heads of alternative practitioners.

This same media mentality has ignored the startling truth about pesticides and the inability of our regulatory agencies to function. Consequently, you will read Congressional testimony in these pages rather than those of the nation's best newspapers.

In addition to the bad news, in this issue we will paint the opposite scenario. We will provide a sound rationale for promoting the growth of an alternate system: an eco-agriculture, a sustainable agriculture, whose most recognizable and supportable form is accessible to the consumer in the rapidly growing infant known as the "organic" farming and food production industry.

And in our next issue we will show that, while much under-investigated, there is a growing body of evidence which strongly suggests that certain of the organic methods of agriculture can indeed produce foods with measurably higher nutrient contents. Not only is organic food free from poison, but it is more vital, and imparts health as no chemically grown foods can possibly do.

The great Dr. Gerson was unafraid to make strong statements, even when he knew that they would evoke controversy. His language was clear, precise, and unequivocal. It is likely that the combined sciences will soon echo his visionary language of 1958:

"We must conclude from these observations that unless the soil is cared for properly, the depleted soil with its abnormal external metabolism will bring about more and more abnormalities of our internal metabolism, resulting in serious degenerative diseases in animals and human beings. The soil needs activity - the natural cycle of growth; it needs protection from erosion; and finally, it needs less and less artificial fertilizer, but more and more of the use of organic waste material in the correct way, to maintain the soil's productivity and life. Food produced in that way - we have to eat as living substances, partly fresh and partly freshly prepared, for life begets life. Organic gardening food seems to be the answer to the cancer problem.

Nutrition labeling is bad for your health

by Gar Hildenbrand

(Excerpted from the Gerson Healing Newsletter, Vol. 5, No. 1, 1989)

I was asked recently by the editor of a proposed new scholarly quarterly to prepare an article discussing the historical beginnings of the Recommended Dietary Allowances (RDAs) and to compare their contemporary uses to the purposes for which their originators created them. In the process of creating an outline for the piece, I read thousands of pages from hundreds of articles dating from the 1800's through to the present.

RDAs were developed to cope with the changes caused by World War II. Normal food supplies were disrupted, new food supplies were available, large groups of people were being assembled in new locations. They were also created to feed our soldiers and our civilian defense workers the "best" possible nutrition: nutrition not simply to provide essentials for survival, but supernutrition to produce better fighters and a stronger nation.

To do this, RDAs were intended to be used as measures of the quality of whole foods, the "protective foods", fruits, vegetables, whole grains, and dairy, which had been long associated in the medical literature with disease resistance, immunity, and physical prowess. Suitability of new crops for consumption was to be determined by testing samples for known nutritional factors (e.g.; vitamins). This Is almost directly analogous to an old time riverboat navigator calling off depth readings. The "go ahead" reading was "mark twain". Just as there is much more to a river than the measurement of a point at which its waters are deep enough to navigate, the RDA originators recognized that there is much more to whole foods than the known nutrients.

Furthermore, RDAs were intended to identify nourishing whole foods to be purchased in massive quantities for groups, not for individuals. They were never intended to tell any individual how much of any vitamin should be taken, nor were they intended to provide manufacturers formulae to "enrich" processed foods.

The savvy consumer should stop reading labels for "Vitamin content." Food constituents thought to be valuable in the prevention of cancer are not even mentioned in the RDAs. Consumers should eat according to the dietary guidelines offered in this issue of the Healing Newsletter. Enriched manufactured or processed foods will never be the nutritional equivalent of whole foods. Consumers should wisely go to the organic produce section, bypassing the boxed, bagged, and canned foods. Let us not be a nation of malnourished, vitamin-wise idiots savants.

Pesticides: How big is the problem?

by Gar Hildenbrand

(Excerpted from the Gerson Healing Newsletter, Vol. 5, No. 1, 1989)

The U.S. food supply is awash in a sea of pesticide formulations. Some of our crops are so thoroughly and repeatedly drenched with poisons and solvents that they could practically float to produce warehouses like logs down a river of chemicals.

It is a familiar umbrage of doubt and suspicion which I cast on pesticides and their manufacturers. Excellent commentaries on the subject have been recently written by Lawrie Mott and Karen Snyder of the National Resources Defense Council ("Pesticide Alert", 1987), Pete Price of the Assembly Office of Research for the State of California ('The Invisible Diet", 1988), and the Committee on Scientific and Regulatory Issues Underlying Pesticide Use Patterns and Agricultural Innovation of the Board on Agriculture of the National Research Council of the National Academy of Sciences ("Regulating Pesticides in Food: The Delaney Paradox", 1987).

Based on the prior labors of Dr. Max Gerson, M.D., the Gerson Institute's involvement with, and vocal opposition to, chronic pesticide abuse is as old as the pesticide industry itself. Since early in the first half of this century, Gerson advocated organic enrichment of food crop bearing soil and avoidance of chronic chemical applications to food crops. In a 1985 speech before the History Division of the American Chemical Society, Albert Einstein College of Medicine Professor of Surgery and Biochemistry Dr. Eli Seifter recalled Gerson's Senate Testimony of 1945.

In his address, entitled "The Contributions of Dr. Max Gerson to Nutritional Chemistry", professor Seifter reviewed Gerson's advocacy of both the disease preventive and therapeutic use of fresh fruits and vegetables grown without DDT and Chlordane. Gerson also warned that crops treated with pesticides should not be consumed.

At that time, according to Seifter, Gerson was ridiculed by members of the American Cancer Society and the U.S. Public Health Services. However, since that time, the American Cancer Society has adopted Gerson's dietary recommendations (with the notable exception of pesticide avoidance, and without credit to Gerson), and both DDT and Chlordane, now known to be carcinogenic, have been banned for food application in the United States.

If Gerson's early warnings were vindicated, why did our national policy makers not act to prevent further abuses and to protect Americans from other chemical threats? What is the history of the U.S. Government's involvement in the regulation of pest control poisons?

Apparently, the majority of legislators did not view pesticides as a problem. Perhaps they simply accepted the manufacturers' empty assurance, "It washes off".

The U.S. Federal Insecticide Act has been a matter of law since 1910. But 'it was not designed to protect consumers against contaminated food. Instead, it was intended by Congress to protect farmers against fraudulent promotions of adulterated pesticides. At that time, many arsenic compounds were used which were later proven to have terrible health consequences and were subsequently banned in the U.S.

The concept of residual chemicals found in the food supply was not a matter of concern in Washington for nearly thirty years.

Although a 1938 Amendment to the Federal Food, Drug, and Cosmetic Act (FDCA) first reflected concern for consumers by addressing tolerance levels for pesticide residues, pesticides were not regulated for consumer protection, for practical purposes, until 1947. The vehicle for regulation which was passed in 1947 was a very weak Federal Insecticide, Fungicide, and Rodenticide Act (FIFRA) which required registration through the U.S. Department of Agriculture (USDA).

FIFRA was so weak that the USDA was impotent. Even if USDA considered an applicant's pesticide hazardous, the manufacturer could obtain a so-called "protest registration" to keep the pesticide on the market. Unbelievably, U.S. taxpayers were obliged to eat probable poisons and to pay for U.S. Government sponsored testing to prove them dangerous before they could be removed from the market.

Sixteen years from the introduction of the concept of food tolerances, the 1954 "Miller Amendment" to FDCA, at last, required FDA to prove pesticides effective and to set tolerances on raw foods.

Public awareness of the problem of pesticides in food was stimulated by the 1962 publication of Rachel Carson's powerful "Silent Spring". Within less than two years, the 1964 Amendments to FIFRA put an end to "protest registration" of hazardous pesticides. Substantial modification of FIFRA also sharply curtailed pesticide manufacturing industries' ability to promulgate chemicals which would injure life forms other than the intended targets.

In 1970, as part of something called "Reorganization Plan #3", the Environmental Protection Agency was put in charge of FIFRA. EPA is still in charge of registering pesticides and setting tolerances.

The Federal Environmental Pesticide Control Act (FEPCA) of 1972 was created under the banner of consumer protection, but actually accomplished quite the opposite. This piece of legislation cast in concrete the abstract, scientifically unsound assumption that chronic pesticide use brought with it a benefit great enough to offset harm to the consumer.

The unfortunate language of FEPCA compels the EPA to register a pesticide if "when used in accordance with widespread and commonly accepted practice, it will not cause unreasonable adverse effects on man or the environment, taking into account the economic, social and environmental costs and benefits of the use of any pesticide".

Assuming that the diseases caused by pesticides will be birth defects, frank mutations, neurological damage, immune incompetence, and cancer, to name a few, we must ask: When is it "reasonable" to cause these diseases in even one person?

These man-made, one might even say industrially sponsored, and so-called "reasonable" diseases of humankind and the environment are altogether abominable; the more so with our knowledge of the rational and forward thinking return to economically, socially, and environmentally successful low input (read low chemical) sustainable agriculture bellwethered by the unsung heroes of America, our independent farmers.

Scientists are currently unable to predict the carcinogenic, mutagenic, and/or teratogenic risks inherent in chronic exposures to low levels of dozens and dozens of probably interactive chemicals. There are far too many variables. Funding for epidemiology is worse than inadequate, and no one thanks a researcher for doing the work.

But our federal laws command EPA to find that known and suspected dangers of chemicals in our food and environment are balanced by short term gains in limited segments of the economy. Metaphorically, EPA has been ordered to go to Heaven by hopping aboard a Hell-bound handbasket.

My critics might argue that I am mistaken regarding the legislative intent and effect of FIFRA, so I hasten to point out that FIFRA required EPA to purchase unsafe pesticides in order to remove them from the market. EPA has compensated offending manufacturers with at least $20 million already. Would a Congress interested in protecting the consumer have forced taxpayers to support the manufacture of suspected poisons?

This practice would have continued had not the recent Congress moved to place the majority of financial burden on the chemical manufacturers instead of the taxpayer. In late 1988, Congress amended FIFRA to require manufacturers to contribute to the toxicological evaluation of their chemicals which had gained registration before current testing criteria had been developed. Under the new law, firms will be assessed fees from $50 thousand up to $150 thousand.

The 1988 legislation also established a nine year deadline for completion by EPA of reviews and evaluation of toxic health risks of pesticides, some of which have been in use for decades now. In 1972, EPA was ordered to review and evaluate some 400 active pesticide ingredients. None of those studies have been completed as of the date of publication of this issue of Healing-

The apparent progress of the above legislation was dealt a stunning setback on October 12, 1988, when the EPA announced an end to a 30-year ban on carcinogenic pesticides known to concentrate in juicing and cooking of fruits and vegetables. EPA's rationale for this anti-consumer/pro-industry move was that it had adopted a "negligible risk" policy developed by the National Academy of Sciences.

In this writer's opinion, EPA is wrong to characterize the "negligible risk" scenario of NAS as a scientific recommendation. EPA chose one of four scenarios NAS offered in an attempt to consider both the purely scientific issues involved in chronic pesticide use and the confusing socioeconomic concept of "balancing" human health risks against perceived economic benefits.

The four NAS scenarios depicted a range of options which included, allow me to stress this, a complete ban of all oncogenic chemical applications to food. EPA was free to choose that option, and a similar "zero-risk" scenario which focused on residues in processed foods. NAS did not, and could not, tell EPA what to do. EPA's directors decided to deregulate carcinogenic pesticides.

EPA was wrong to do this.

But that is where we stand today. Chemicals have been sanctioned by the U.S. Government at levels considered unreasonable and unsafe by many experts. That is not to say that there is harmony in the government regarding these issues.

The fur is flying at EPA and FDA. During April of 1987, the powerful Chairman John Dingell of the U.S. House of Representatives' Energy and Commerce Committee (which controls the budgets for the National Institutes of Health) held grueling hearings into what Dingell characterized as "serious deficiencies in the Federal pesticide monitoring program". The hearings were held by the Energy and Commerce Subcommittee on Oversight and Investigations. Representatives Waxman, Sikorski, Wyden and others joined the Hon. Mr. Dingell, who also chairs the Subcommittee, in a roast of the FDA and its Commissioner Frank Young.

Why has the national press remained silent on these investigations? We are certain that our readers will want to know what is being said and done, and by whom. So, we are certain, should readers of the New York Times, the Washington Post, the LA Times, the Des Moines Register, and others. Readers, why not write your local press corps and inquire regarding their lack of knowledge/interest in this subject? Perhaps you might stimulate them to look into 'it.

As the hearings opened, the Honorable Mr. Henry Waxman, U.S. Representative from California, spoke pointedly saying, "The American people want to believe that our food, whether produced here or abroad, is free from unsafe pesticide residues. They want to believe that our Government is doing all that is necessary to protect them. The record compiled to date by EPA and FDA leaves me with little confidence that the public is getting what it wants and deserves. The most generous characterization of our current situation is, simply put, we just don't know if our food is safe.

"How can we be in this intolerable predicament? The Federal Food, Drug, and Cosmetic Act mandates that EPA allow pesticide residues to remain on food only if they are safe to consume. Yet, according to testimony by EPA before the Subcommittee on Health and Environment last summer, EPA has complete scientific data for approximately 10 percent of the food-use pesticides currently being applied to our crops. Most pesticides still face years of additional testing before EPA will have the necessary data to make a regulatory decision.

"In addition, EPA can only speculate about the safety of many of the inactive ingredients used in pesticides and about the metabolites and breakdown products of the currently used active ingredients. The bottom line is that EPA approved pesticide residue levels are outdated and unsupported by scientific data.* Yet, farmers apply pesticides every day with the intention of staying within these EPA regulatory limits.

"To make a bad situation even worse, we can only hope that our food contains no more than the EPA-set residue levels because the FDA cannot tell us with certainty that our food meets even the inadequate EPA standards."

The Honorable Ron Wyden, U.S. Representative from Oregon, observed in his opening statements that "(T)he U.S. system for inspecting food is a non-system. Imported foods tainted with dangerous pesticides slip by the Food and Drug Administration because virtually none of this food is tested. Rather than protecting the American public, our food inspection system forces Americans to play Russian roulette at the grocery store. All too often, adulterated food is permitted on the shelves of our supermarkets before Food and Drug Administration test results are in.

"When imported food arrives in this country, the Food and Drug Administration inspectors don't sample a fair cross section of that food. Many pesticides found on foods from major exporting countries have been banned or considered serious health hazards in this country. These toxic chemicals have often been overlooked by the Food and Drug Administration.

"The inspectors tend to focus on high volume foods, leaving the low volume foods unexamined. For example, in fiscal years 1983 through 1985, 46 million pounds of raspberries entered our ports and only two samples were collected; 251 million pounds of yams were imported into this country and only 24 samples were taken.

"By the time the Food and Drug Administration discovers a violation, the food usually has been eaten. The FDA doesn't fine the importers and can't fine the growers.

"Who loses in the Russian roulette game? Obviously, the consumer, but often the American farmer, who has to compete against foreign growers who use those chemicals banned in this country."

The most colorful and effective opening remarks were made by the gifted and Honorable Gerry Sikorski, U.S. Representative from Minnesota: "During the last 15 or 20 years, we have learned a great deal about dangerous chemicals in the foods we eat and the beverages we drink. We have had cancer-causing cyclamates in diet soda, EDB's in cake mixes, sulfites in our salad bars, and red dye No. 2 in crimson M&M's.

"The result of all this knowledge has been, or so we thought, a safer diet. Some additives have been banned. Although some dubious ones remained on the market, at least we could act as informed consumers, knowing what foods to avoid. We could always go natural, to fruits and vegetables and such.

"It's spring, and we are pulling out the picnic baskets and, as surely as summer follows spring, a sequel to "Jaws" follows the Sports Illustrated swimsuit edition. And now, just when we thought it was safe to go back into the grocery store, it turns out that the safest waters, our fresh fruits and vegetables, have become infested with angry chemical sharks.

"Our regulatory lifeguard, the FDA, has known about the presence of these chemicals in imported foods for many years. The American consumer remains an unwary swimmer. We have a pesticide suspected of causing gene mutations, cancer, and birth defects, benomyl, in bananas,"

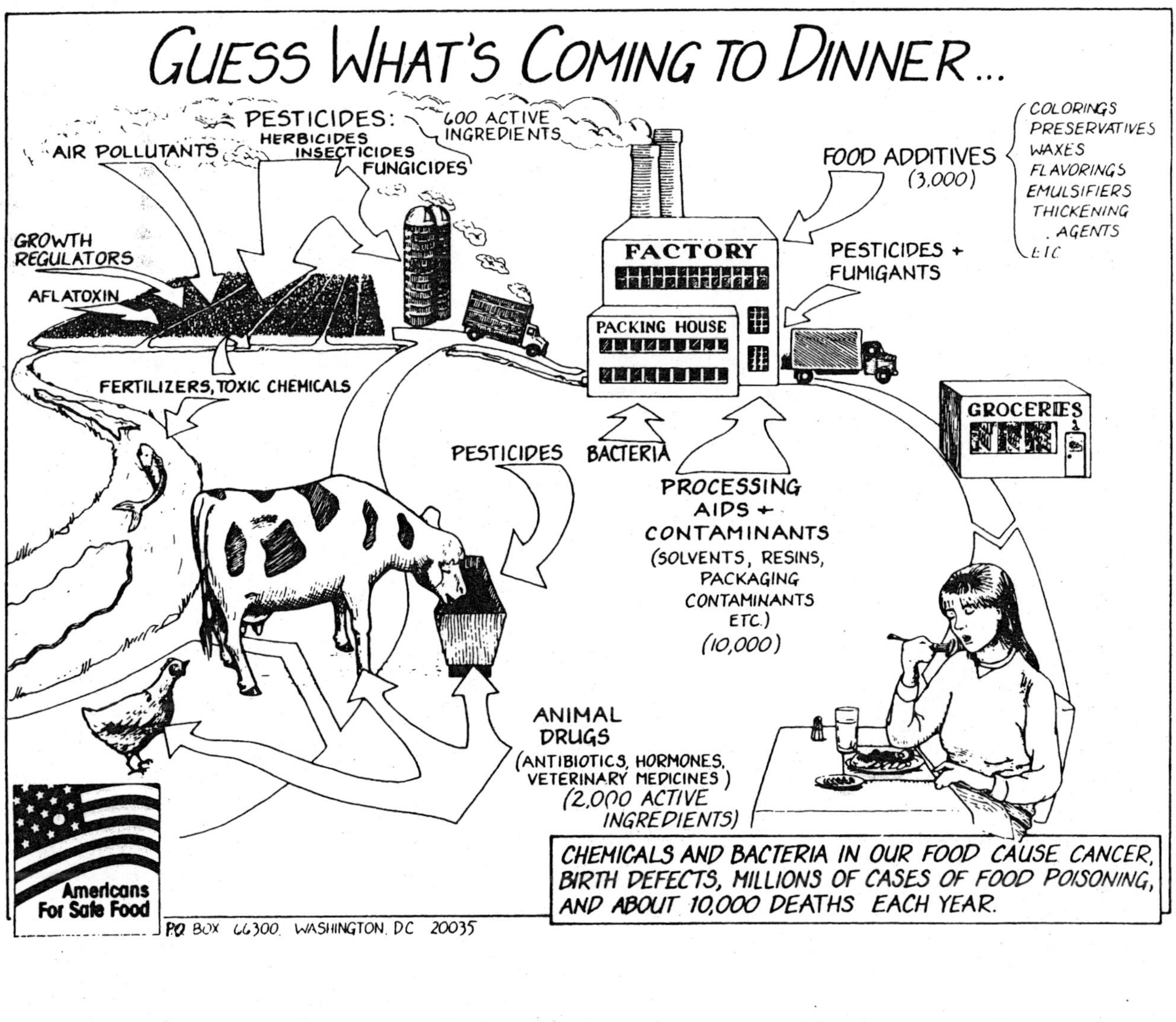

...(here the Congress-man held up a banana for visual effect)..."the single largest fruit imported in the United States. We eat about 6 billion pounds of this each year. And we eat a lot of winter tomatoes in Minnesota,"...(holding a tomato in his other hand)..."which we have always thought tasted like flavored Styrofoam strip-mined in some strange foreign southern clime, and now we find they may well contain EBDC's, an acknowledged carcinogen.

"The FDA hasn't tested a single Mexican tomato for EBDC's and has in 8 years only tested 2 bananas for benomyl out of 50 to 60 billion pounds of them. The list of hazardous fruits and vegetables and pesticide residues goes on.

"In study after study by this subcommittee, the FDA, and the GAO (General Accounting Office), problems have been identified with FDA's testing program and steps have been recommended to address the problem, but instead of action, we hear the same excuse from FDA that we hear from so many of our Federal regulatory agencies - not the Pentagon - under this administration. They say, we don't have the resources and, yes there may be a problem, but we make do with what we have. We hear a lot about getting the Government off our backs from the same people who are content to have more carcinogens in our children's blood streams.

'The fact is FDA can't make do with what it has. To protect the public health and safety, it needs better data systems, more efficient targeting of hazardous pesticides and tougher enforcement. The FDA can no longer be bashful about hazardous food imports. The time has arrived to subject the Chiquita banana lady to a serious strip search at our borders."

The Honorable Rick Boucher, U.S. Representative from Virginia, pointed out "that despite the results of a number of in-house and independent investigations, which have pointed with alarm to the inadequacies of FDA's food testing and enforcement programs, that the Agency receives a failing grade for its efforts to ensure that our food provides nutrition and not the chemical catalysts of chronic illness.

"The purpose of today's hearing is to uncover, as best we can, the foundation of that failure. Is it a lack of resources? Is it a lack of commitment? Or perhaps is it some underlying insensitivity to the real health threats posed by pesticides for which the EPA has established tolerance levels?"

California U.S. Representative Leon Panetta, of the Committee on Agriculture, observed that "about 26 percent of the food product that goes to our consumers" comes from abroad, much of it containing "pesticides that in some instances have been outlawed in this country for 10 years".

Calling the pesticide problem "a time bomb that's there and ready to go off", Congressman Panetta proclaimed, "It's a situation that cannot be tolerated. It is unfair: it is unsafe."

Assistant Comptroller General Dexter Peach of the Resources, Community, and Economic Development Division of the General Accounting Office (GAO) summarized GAO's recent reports on the EPA's re-registration and tolerance setting process and the FDA's monitoring programs for both domestic and imported foods. His points were compelling.

• FDA relies on tests which miss approximately 50% of the pesticides currently in use, including identified high-health-risk chemicals.

• FDA does not know, even though the information is available, what pesticides are used on imported produce, and therefore usually does not test for them.

• FDA frequently does not remove even identified adulterated foods from the market in the relatively few instances when it does detect them. 60% of identified adulterated domestic food was consumed by the American public. The minimum estimate of identified adulterated imported food consumed by Americans is 45%.

• FDA normally does not fine companies which are found to be selling contaminated food. Action was taken against only 10% of offenders in cases reviewed.

• FDA statistics for 40 selected foods imported into the U.S. revealed that foods from some of the importing countries were not sampled, some for as long as six years.

• FDA failed, during a three year period for which GAO had records, to test pineapples from 17 of 26 importing countries, including the major importer of pineapples. FDA failed entirely to test pineapples from eight of those countries for six calendar years, even though data revealed illegal residues on nearly 20% of the pineapples tested.

• Gaps exist in understanding the

health risks associated with many pesticides.

• EPA lacks the data with which to determine safe residue limits for many pesticides.

• EPA lacks data regarding health hazards of "inert" pesticide formula ingredients, such as solvents like 2-methoxyethanol which has been shown to produce adverse reproductive, and developmental toxicity, effects in lab animals. (There are about 1,200 "inert" ingredients in approximately 50,000 pesticide formulations).

• EPA lacks data regarding health hazards of pesticides in groundwater. Minimal groundwater testing has identified 17 pesticide chemicals. 70 currently used pesticides are suspected of being capable of leaching into groundwaters.

• Existing tolerances for 390 of the 400 pesticide chemicals now registered were set without all the data EPA now believes is necessary to assess health risks according to current scientific standards.

• EPA, at the rate it is moving, cannot possibly complete registration and tolerance reassessment of the 390 incompletely documented chemicals in less than 20-30 years.

Accompanying Mr. Peach was National Resources Defense Council Senior Scientist, Lawrie Mott. Along with colleague Karen Snyder, Ms. Mott written "Pesticide Alert" which was published last year. Ms. Mott is a molecular biochemist, trained at Yale University.

In her testimony Ms. Mott explained, "Often tolerances are established (by EPA) without sufficient toxicological data to assure that the levels chosen are safe (or human exposure. In some cases when data do exist, they are inadequate, invalid, or even fabricated.

"Further, when developing tolerances EPA has relied on arbitrary assumptions about what constitutes an average diet, and what safety factors should be used. Tolerances are rarely revised when new scientific information is received about a pesticide. Inert ingredients and other chemicals of toxicological concerns such as metabolites or break-down products that may leave residues in food are not considered in tolerances.

"Many pesticide tolerances were established without information on the chemical's potential to cause cancer, birth defects, sterility or genetic mutation. For example, by the end of fiscal year 1985, EPA had reviewed tolerances for 117 active ingredients through their registration standards program. Only four registration standards identified tolerances as adequate and fully supported by the necessary health and safety data. Fourteen registration standards revealed that the public's maximum potential exposure to the pesticide in food may exceed the amount considered safe to ingest.

"For instance, EPA calculated that the maximum potential dietary exposure to the insecticide lindane exceeds the acceptable daily intake by 7,883 percent. Forchlorpyrifos, ethion and endosulfan, pesticides found commonly in food, the potential human exposure exceeded the acceptable daily intake by 313 percent, 258 percent, and 140 percent, respectively.

"For 23 other chemicals, the registration standards indicated that EPA had insufficient data to determine the amount of residues considered safe to ingest. Nonetheless, these chemicals are continuing to be used on food.

"Another issue rendering EPA's tolerance setting system ineffective is the complete failure to regulate the inert ingredients contained in pesticide products.

"Recently, EPA reviewed the 1,200 commonly used inerts to identify the chemicals of toxicological concern. As a result, the Agency developed two lists of approximately 100 inert ingredients that present human health risks.

"List one contained inerts of toxicological concern, and list two contained the inerts that are potentially toxic based on structural similarities to compounds already known to be hazardous.

"(The National Resources Defense Council) has learned that at least 30 of these pernicious inerts have received exemptions from tolerances...These exempted chemicals that may be occurring as residues in our food include the carcinogens benzene, epichlorohydrin, formaldehyde, methylene chloride, and vinyl chloride.

"At best, FDA's five scans can cumulatively detect approximately 40 percent of the chemicals that may leave residues in our food. Some of these chemicals that cannot be detected include the dangerous pesticides benomyl, daminozide, the EBDC's, paraquat, DBCP, and dinoseb. In fact, approximately 40 percent of all the pesticides classified by FDA as having a moderate to high health hazard cannot be detected by any of the five multiresidue scans."

Ms. Mott stated strongly a point with which the Gerson Institute fully agrees, "Due to the numerous weaknesses in EPA's tolerances that I discussed earlier, the public cannot assume that only residues in excess of tolerances are dangerous. Between the fiscal years 1982 and 1985. FDA analyzed approximately 20,000 samples of 26 kinds of commonly consumed fruits and vegetables. Pesticide residues were detected in 48 percent of all the foods monitored. And this number probably understates the extent of pesticide residues in our food because the FDA's routine methods for detecting chemicals only detect about half of the chemicals used on our foods."

One particularly revealing moment occurred during an exchange between Rep. Wyden and Mr. Kevin Donohue, group director from GAO. Rep. Wyden had asked whether there were holes in the Total Diet Study, or Market Basket

Study. In 1983, FDA Associate Commissioner Joseph Hile had haled it as "effective in showing over the years that the American consumer's dietary exposure to pesticide residues has been consistently below acceptable limits of exposure set by the World Health Organization". After issuance of a critical GAO report in 1986, Secretary Bowen claimed that the Total Diet Study showed that "the U.S. consumer is not being exposed to harmful levels of pesticide residues".

Mr. Donohue responded: "What they do in the Total Diet Study is that they take a market basket from various grocery stores in different parts of the country. This is done four times a year in four different parts of the country. Then they run the food through a series of tests. From the information available to us, the same problems we found in FDA's pesticide monitoring program exist in the Total Diet Study. That is, heavy reliance on the multiresidue test.

"For instance, the records according to FDA files, show that the EBDC is not tested in the Total Diet Study.

"One of the other things is that they have made some improvements since 1979. At that time, they were targeting three age groups. Currently they are targeting eight. For instance, maybe the majority of the people on the subcommittee today are not covered by that. In other words, the category of people 31 to 59 is not covered."

Rep. Wyden asked, "Am I to understand that the coverage of the Total Diet Study excludes the high health hazard pesticides which are not covered by multiresidue methods, such as the EBDC's?"

"That's right," said Mr. Donohue, "they have not tested EBDC's at all."

Rep. Sikorski, the colorful speaker who had earlier displayed tomatoes and bananas, offered an important observation, "I think it's important to remember that what we're talking about are not things that show up on the outside. If you peel this banana, you're not free from the problem. It's in the actual meat. When you peel the banana, you're just getting to the problem. When you eat the tomato, you can wash it in the sink, which you should do, but we're talking about systemic compounds whose residues are within the food itself."

Shortly afterward, biochemist Mott added, "(S)ome chemicals will penetrate, no matter how they are applied, they will translocate. Other chemicals, if you apply them late in the growing season, will only be on the surface, whereas if you apply them in the early season they will penetrate the entire fruit.

'The other problem is that even if the residues are limited to the surface, many chemicals are designed not to be water-soluble, because (pesticide manufacturers) don't want them to wash off the plant in the field. (They) want to have the effect on the target. So washing won't even remove residues that may be limited to the surface.

"What consumers should do is they should try to buy locally grown produce in season. They may want to avoid food that is shipped great distances that could have been treated to prevent spoilage during travel. And also, I would recommend that consumers ask their supermarkets if they can stock organically grown food.

"For example, all 125 Safeway stores in the United Kingdom sell organically grown produce. There is organically grown produce available in varying degrees throughout our Nation, and the food industry should consider marketing it along with commercial produce."

The Gerson Institute joins with the National Resources Defense Council in urging consumers to purchase organically grown foods. Consumers should step out of the role of the unwitting or unwilling victim. Stop relying on the U.S. Government to force the pesticide industry to change. We must make the changes ourselves. The U.S. government must follow the will of the people. And industry cannot sell chemically grown and poisonous produce to people who will not buy it. Don't buy it!

Glossary:

ACTIVE INGREDIENT: An ingredient in a pesticide product that destroys or controls a pest.

CARCINOGEN: A substance or mixture of substances that produces or incites cancer in a living tissue.

FUNGICIDE: Chemicals used to kill or suppress the growth of all fungi or a certain fungus (mushrooms, molds, mildews, rusts, etc).

HERBICIDE: A class of pesticide used to kill or suppress the growth of all or a certain type of plant.

ILLEGAL RESIDUE: The presence of an active ingredient in ammounts above the tolerance on a crop at harvest. In some cases, any amount of chemical present on the crop is considered illegal if no tolerance exists for the pesticide on the commodity.

INERT INGREDIENT: A substance contained in a pesticide product or formulation that is not intended to kill or control the target pest but rather used to dissolve, dilute, propel, or stabilize the active ingredient in the pesticide product.

INSECTICIDE: A class of pesticide that prevents, destroys, repels or mitigates insects.

MUTAGEN: A substance or agent that produces genetic changes in living cells.

ONCOGENICITY: The tendency for the development of tumors in organisms exposed to a chemical substance.

PERSISTENT PESTICIDES: Pesticides that remain in the environment and do not degrade or metabolize to innocuous constituents for months or perhaps years.

PESTICIDE: A general term (or chemical or biological products used to destroy pests; (unwanted) insects, plants, fungi, rodents, bacteria, or other organisms.

REGISTRATION: Licenses for specified uses of pesticide products. A pesticide product registration sets the terms and conditions of the use that the product, including the directions and precautions for use outlined on the product label. All pesticides must be registered by EPA before they can be sold to the public.

REREGISTRATION: A reassessment of previously registered pesticides according to current scientific standards.

SYNERGISM: The tendency of chemicals acting in combination to produce effects greater than the sum of the effects of the individual chemicals.

TOLERANCE: The maximum amount of pesticide residue that is legally permitted in a food. EPA sets a distinct residue limit for each individual food to which the pesticide may be applied.

TOXICITY: The harmful effects produced by a chemical.

A Coffee Enema? Now I've Heard Everything.

The Coffee Enema: What does it do?, how does it work?

by Gar Hildenbrand

(Excerpted from the Gerson Healing Newsletter #13, May-June 1989)

It is difficult to describe the incredulous facial expressions which ripple across a medical school lecture audience as the topic of coffee enemas is introduced. Embarrassed sniggering is heard from several seats in the hall.

A wise guy heckles, "How do you take it?" Charlotte Gerson doesn't miss a beat, answering "Black - without cream and sugar." Laughter relaxes the entire room and Gerson goes on to explain this aspect of her famous father's (Max Gerson, M.D.) treatment: 3 tablespoons of drip-grind coffee, boiled in a quart of distilled water for 3 minutes, covered and simmered for 15 minutes, cooled to body temperature, filtered, and admitted to the colon using a 6-8" tip while lying on the right side. This is held for 12-15 minutes and released.

Responses from the audience are typical: "Boy, I'll bet you get a buzz out of that!" "Couldn't you just drink three or four cups of coffee?"

And the eventual "big question" is "What does it do?" "Why go to all that trouble just for a caffeine high?"

The coffee enema is, without question, the most unusual part of Gerson's combined regime (1), and often evokes astonishment and mirth in persons who have never experienced an enema and who emphatically prefer to drink their coffee. Practitioners and patients who have had experience with coffee enemas, however, know that they are far more than a means of introducing stimulating caffeine into the bloodstream. From the patient's point of view, the coffee enema means relief from depression, confusion, general nervous tension, many allergy related symptoms and, most importantly, relief from severe pain.

In 1981, writing in Medical Hypotheses (2), Mark F. McCarty pointed out that "At a Senate Select Subcommittee hearing on cancer research in 1946 (3), five independent M.D.s who had had personal experience with patients treated by Gerson, submitted letters indicating that they had been surprised and encouraged by the results they had seen, and urged a widespread trial of the method (4). One of these doctors claimed that relief of severe pain was achieved in about 90% of cases. No controlled trial of Gerson's methods has ever been undertaken."

The coffee enema has a very specific purpose: lowering serum toxins. Dr. Peter Lechner, who conducted a trial of the Gerson cancer therapy in the post-surgical treatment of liver-metastasized colorectal cancers under the aegis of the Landes-krankenhaus of Graz, Austria, reported (5) in 1984 "Coffee enemas have a definite effect on the colon which can be observed with an endoscope. Wattenberg and coworkers were able to prove in 1981 that the palmitic acid found in coffee promotes the activity of glutathione S-transferase and other ligands by manyfold times above the norm. It is this enzyme group which is responsible primarily for the conjugation of free electrophile radicals which the gall bladder will then release."

The importance of this action of coffee enemas is best described against the background of modern concepts of cell ion and water content.

In most, probably all, chronic degenerative diseases there exists a "tissue damage syndrome" first described by Cope (6). When cells are challenged by poison, oxygen starvation, malnutrition, or trauma (a physical blow), a uniform set of reactions takes place: cells a) lose potassium, b) accept excess sodium and chloride, and c) swell with excess water.

According to the work of Ling, recently summarized in his monograph "In Search of the Physical Basis of Life" (Ling, G.N., Plenum Press, New York, 1984), the cellular cytoplasm is latticed with a protein-lipid macromolecule through which an electron current flows. Energy-storing adenosine triphosphate (ATP), the main product of metabolism, is complexed with this macromolecule, polarizing and energizing it, and forming many interactive, cooperative association sites which prefer potassium over sodium.

In a resting, healthy cell with sufficient ATP, water is highly organized in polarized multiple layers forming an "ice-like" structure. Water and ice are different not because their molecules are different, but because their molecules relate differently.

According to Ling's Association-Induction Hypothesis, being "alive" requires not only the presence of the right composition of chemical compounds, but also requires that they be maintained in special electronic and steric (atomic spatial) relationships. The living state is a high energy state in the same sense as a cocked gun, a drawn bow, or a set mousetrap.

In the living cell, potassium and nearly all water (except that in vacuoles, etc.) is in an adsorbed state. Potassium is preferentially adsorbed on the beta- and gamma- carboxyl groups of certain cellular proteins while water is adsorbed in polarized multilayers on a matrix of extended protein chains. Low levels of sodium in the cell are due to the reduced solubility of structured water. This mechanism also contains water content.

Cope reasoned that challenge to the cell by toxins, oxygen starvation, malnutrition, or trauma will result in an altered molecular configuration state in which the macromolecule will lose its preference for potassium. Sodium competes with potassium for association sites In damaged cells.

Loss of cell potassium and increase of cell sodium in turn results in decreased electron flow through the macromolecule. This in turn causes decreased attraction of paramagnetic ions and subsequent disorganization of water molecules. Because bulk phase water, structured in a high-energy state, is the main mechanism controlling cell water content and purity, any disturbance in water structuring will result in the cell swelling with excess water and extracellular solutes.

Once the internal environment of the cell is polluted with excess water and extracellular materials, mitochondrial production of ATP is greatly impaired with the result that cells cannot produce sufficient energy to repair themselves unless the challenge is removed.

Endogenous serum toxins can be generated by cells with impaired metabolism, by bacteria, and by malignant cells. NMR studies have suggested that surrounding active malignancies there may often be a sphere of damaged normal tissue in which water structuring is impaired by the chronic insult of tumor toxins. Energy production and immunity are depressed in these cells which are swollen with excess salt and water. Such damaged tissue has decreased circulation because oversized edematous cells crowd arterioles, capillaries, and lymph ducts.

Gerson taught that improved circulation and tissue integrity would prevent spread and, in fact, cause the destruction of malignant tumors. He held as axiomatic the observation that no cancer could exist in normal metabolism. A favorite example of his was the well known resistance of healthy lab models to tumor transplants. Such transplanted tumors are quickly killed in many cases by inflammation in the healthy host. In order to cause transplanted tumors to "take" easily, it is necessary to impair the metabolism of the host by damaging the thyroid and adrenal glands. Gerson's efforts were directed toward creating a near normal metabolism in tissues surrounding tumors.

Such protective liver and gut enzyme systems are probably enhanced many fold by coffee enemas. Editors of Physiological Chemistry and Physics stated (7) "Caffeine enemas cause dilation of bile ducts, which facilitates excretion of toxic cancer breakdown products by the liver and dialysis of toxic products from blood across the coionic wall."

Enzyme systems in the liver and small bowel are responsible for conversion and neutralization of the most common tissue toxins, polyamines, ammonia, toxic-bound nitrogen, and electrophiles, all of which can cause cell and membrane damage.

In the late 1970's and early 1980s, researchers in the lab of Lee Wattenberg (8-13) identified salts of palmitic acids (kahweol and cafestol palmitate) in coffee as potent enhancers of glutathione S-transferase, a major detoxification system that catalyzes the binding of a vast variety of electrophiles from the blood stream to the sulfhydryl group of glutathione. Because the reactive ultimate carcinogenic forms of chemicals are electrophiles, the glutathione S-transferase system must be regarded as an important mechanism for carcinogen detoxification. In mice, this system is enhanced 600% in the liver and 700% in the small bowel when coffee beans are added to their diet. Because this system in lab models is close, if not directly analogous, to that of humans a parallel stimulation by coffee of glutathione S-transferase in humans is probable.

With this rationale in mind, we can expand on Gerson's hypothesized physiological actions and effects of coffee enemas. Gerson wrote that Heubner and Meyer of Geottingen University, Germany, had shown in animal models that rectal administration of caffeine would dilate bile ducts and promote bile flow. The introduction of a quart of coffee solution into the colon will dilute portal blood and, subsequently, the bile. Theophylline and theobromine, major constituents of coffee, dilate blood vessels and counter inflammation of the gut. The palmitates of coffee enhance glutathione S-transferase which is responsible for the removal of many toxic radicals from serum. Finally, the fluid of the enema itself stimulates the visceral nervous system promoting peristalsis and the transit of diluted toxic bile from the duodenum out the rectum. Because the stimulating enema is retained for 15 minutes, and because all the blood in the body passes through the liver nearly every three minutes, these enemas represent a form of dialysis of blood across the gut wall.

It is obvious in light of the above that oral administration of beverage coffee cannot have the same effect. On the contrary, it virtually insures reabsorption of toxic bile.

As a medication, the coffee enema is in a class by itself. While other agents classed as choleretics do increase bile flow from the liver, they do little to enhance detoxifying enzyme systems, and they do not ensure the passage of bile from the intestines out the rectum. Bile is normally reabsorbed up to 9 or 10 times before working its way out the intestines in feces. The enzyme enhancing ability of the coffee enema is unique among choleretics. Because it does not allow reabsorption of toxic bile by the liver across the gut wall, it is an entirely effective means of detoxifying the blood stream through existing enzyme systems in the liver and small bowel. Because clinical practice has shown coffee enemas to be well tolerated by patients when used as frequently as every four hours, the coffee enema may be classed as the only non-reabsorbed, effective, repeatable choleretic in the medical literature.

These enemas are safe when used within the context of the combined regime of Gerson. It is apparent that Gerson's intention in supplying a sodium restricted, high potassium, high micronutrient dietary of fruits, vegetables, and whole grains, was to supply all nutrients, known and unknown, which are necessary for cell respiration and energy production. High potassium, low sodium environments tend to return cell macromolecules to normal configuration states and to improve water structuring and water content. The addition by Gerson of supplemental salts of potassium (acetate, gluconate, and phosphate monobasic) to the diet in which malate is supplied by frequent use of apples probably greatly improves the efficiency of the Kreb's cycle in mitochondrial energy production. Protein restriction, employed by Gerson as a temporary aspect of treatment, has been observed empirically since before the turn of the century to aid in the reduction of cellular edema. Administration of high loading dosages of thyroid and Lugol's solution (iodine and potassium iodide in dilute solution) probably result in multiplication of mitochondria, which have their own DNA and RNA and replicate independently of the cell. Additionally, thyroid is known to enhance cell oxidation of sugars and therefore ATP production. In this way cell energy production is probably markedly increased.

Through these mechanisms, the therapy of Dr. Max Gerson appears to a) reduce serum toxins to eliminate chronic challenge to damaged normal cells, b) improve cell potassium ion content, c) reduce cell sodium content, d) reduce cell swelling through improved water structuring, e) increase cell mitochondria count and activity, and f) supply micronutrients necessary for cell energy production and repair. The contribution of low serum toxin levels by regular administration of coffee enemas is basic to increased cell energy production, enhanced tissue integrity, improved circulation, improved immunity, and improved tissue repair and regeneration which have been observed clinically to result from the administration of the combined regime of Gerson.

References

1. Gerson, M„ 1958. "A Cancer Therapy: Results of Fifty Cases" pp. 190-191(4th Edition, 1986), published by Gerson Institute

2. McCarty, M„ 1981. Medical Hypotheses 7:591-597, "Aldosterone and the Gerson diet - a speculation"

3. Subcommittee of the Committee on Foreign Relations of the United States Senate, 1946, Seventy-ninth Congress, Second Session, Hearings on Bill S.1875, pp. 95-126, United States Government Printing Office, July 1, 2, and 3,1946.

4. ibid, pp. 116-125.

5. Lechner, P., 1984. Proceedings of the Oesterreicher Gesellschaft fur Chirurgie, June 21-23, 1984. "Dietary Regime to be Used in Oncological Postoperative Care."

6. Cope, F.W., 1977. Physiological Chemistry and Physics, 9(6):547-553, 1977. "Pathology of Structured Water and Associated Cations in Cells (The Tissue Damage Syndrome) and its Medical Treatment."

7. Gerson, M„ 1979. Physiological Chemistry and Physics, 10(5): 449-464, 1978. "The Cure of Advanced Cancer by Diet Therapy: a Summary of 30 Years of Clinical Experimentation."

8. Chasseaud, L.F„ 1979. Advanced Cancer Research, 29:175-274, 1979. "The Role of Glutathione S-trans-

ferases in the Metabolism of Chemical Carcinogens and Other Electrophilic Agents."

9. Jakoby, W.B., 1978. Advanced Enzymologyand Related Areas of Molecular Biology, 46:383-414, 1978. "A Group of Multifunctional Detoxification Proteins."

10. Sparnins, V.L; Wattenberg, L.W„ 1981. Journal of the National Cancer Institute, 66:769-771, 1981. "Enhancement of Glutathione S-transferase Activity of the Mouse Forestomach by Inhibitors of Benzo[a]pyrene-induced Neoplasia of Forestomach."

11. Sparnins, V.L., 1980. Proceedings of the American Association of Cancer Researchers and the American Society of Clinical Oncologists, 21:80, Abstract 319. "Effects of Dietary Constituents on Glutathione S-transferase (G-S-T) Activity."

12. Sparnins, V.L.; Lam, L.K.T.; Wattenberg, L.W„ 1981. Proceedings of the American Association of Cancer Researchers and the American Society of Clinical Oncologists, 22:114, Abstract 453. "Effects of Coffee on Glutathione S-transferase (G-S-T) Activity and 7-12-dimethylbenz(a)anthracene (DMBA)- induced Neoplasia."

13. Lam, L.K.T.; Sparnins, V.L.; Wattenberg, L.W„ 1982. Cancer Research, 42:1193-1198, 1982. "Isolation and Identification of Kahweol Palmitate and Cafestol Palmitate as Active Constituents of Green Coffee Beans That Enhance Glutathione S-transferase Activity in the Mouse."

Appendix III: Recipes

These recipes were compiled and edited by Christeene Lindsay-Hildenbrand. To be used in conjunction with the Gerson Therapy videotape: "Charlotte Gerson Demonstrates Basic Gerson Food Preparation."

NOTE: *Recipes marked with * were contributed by Yvonne Nienstadt, Director of Health Services at Cal-a-Vie, Vista, California. Recipes marked with + were contributed by Susan DeSimone of the Gerson Institute. Recipes marked with [MZ] were contributed by Marisol Zuniga of the Hospital Meridien. Recipes marked with [GSG] were contributed by the Gerson Support Group, England. Recipes marked [DAIRY] contain restricted dairy ingredients, instructions on pg. 98 should be followed carefully.*

Gerson Therapy Recipes

Use only certified organically grown fruits, dried fruits, vegetables, grains and sweeteners.
Use fresh fruits and vegetables - no canned.
Fruits and vegetables should not be peeled or scraped unless indicated.
To clean them use only lukewarm water and brush.
Gerson approved light honey, maple syrup and sugar. Dried organic cane sugar (Sucanat®) may be used in recipes calling for brown sugar. It has a strong molasses flavor. Some cooks may prefer other options.

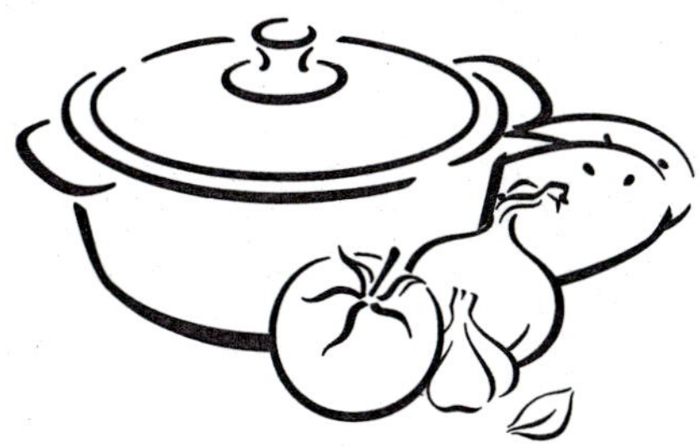

Special Soup

(formerly, Hippocrates Soup)

For 1 person use a 4-quart pot, use the following vegetables, then cover with distilled water:

1 medium celery knob
(substitute 3-4 stalks of celery)
1 medium parsley root
garlic as desired
2 small leeks
1 1/2 lbs. tomatoes or more
2 medium onions
1 lb. potatoes
a little parsley

Do not peel any of these vegetables; just wash and scrub them well and cut them coarsely; simmer them slowly for 2 hours, then put through food mill in small portions; scarcely any fibers should be left. Vary the amount of water used for cooking according to taste and desired consistency. Keep well covered in refrigerator no longer than 2 days. Warm up as much as needed each time.
Note: *For recipes which call for soup stock use the liquid from this special soup.*

Juices

Always freshly prepared. It is impossible to prepare all juices for the day in the morning.

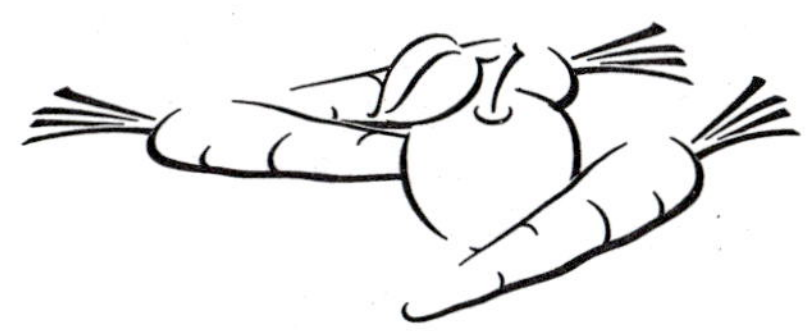

Carrot-Apple

(8 oz. juice)

3 Carrots (6 oz.)
1 Large Green Apple (6 oz.)

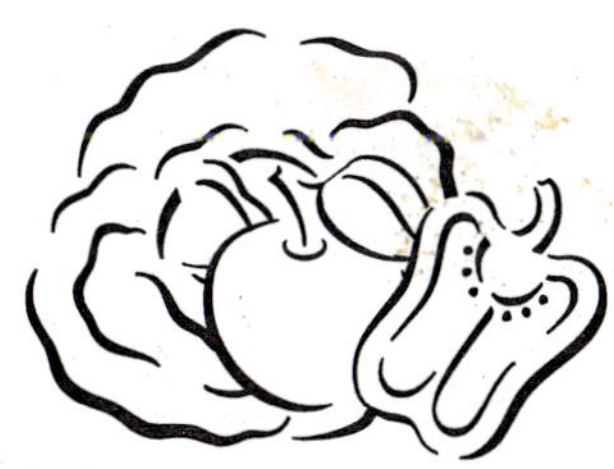

Green Juice

Of the various kinds of leaves mentioned below, procure as many as possible (no others):

Romaine Lettuce
Swiss Chard
Beet Tops (young inner leaves)
Watercress
Some Red Cabbage
Green Pepper (1/4 of small one)
Endive
Escarole

Add one medium apple for each glass when grinding.

Preparation Of Juices
(*A Cancer Therapy*, pg. 240)

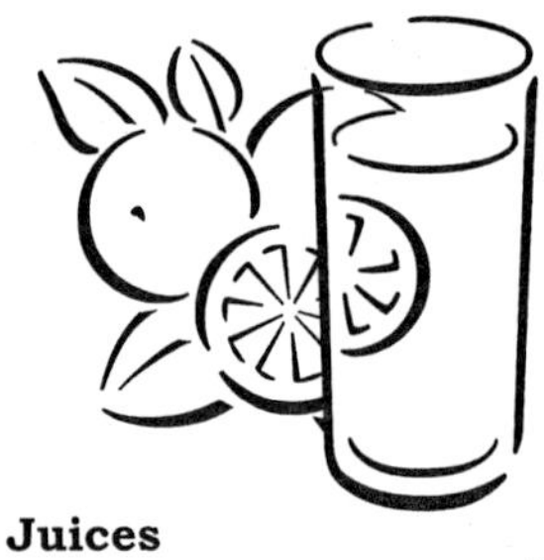

Citrus Juices
Squeeze only with a reamer type juicer made of glass, plastic, porcelain. Do not use any juice press into which the orange is inserted with the skin (if the skin is also pressed out, it will emit harmful fatty acids and aromatic substances contained in its surface). Do not use an aluminum juicer.

Juicers
Use a separate grinder and a separate press. Do not use liquifiers, centrifuges, juice mixers or masters, etc.

Pressing Process
Take 1 or 2 coarsely woven cloths, nylon - 12" square, place cupful of pulp into center of moistened cloth, fold in thirds in both directions and press.
Rinse cloths in cool water after each juice preparation. Do not allow juice to dry on the cloths. Wash thoroughly each night in warm or hot water; rinse thoroughly. Keep overnight in freezer. It is most important to clean machine and cloths very well.
If juice retains taste of cloth, use a new cloth. Allow 2 cloths per juice. Have 1 set of cloths for each type of juice.
Leftovers of all pressings can be used only for compost or as animal food.
If the patient goes to work again, apple and carrot juice only may be taken and kept in a thermos for no longer than 4 hours.

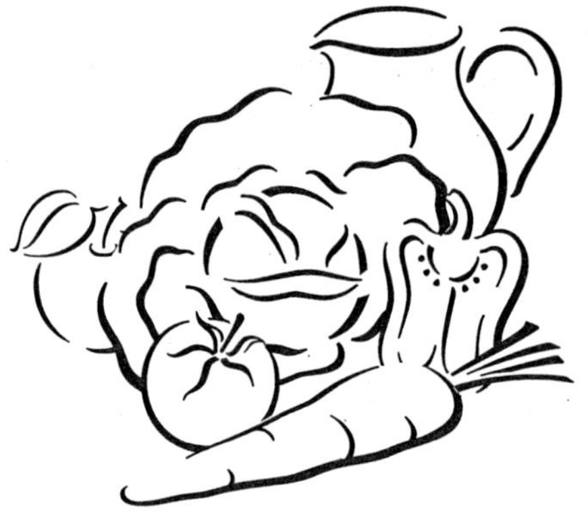

Salads & Dressing
Raw fruit or raw vegetables, when finely grated or shredded, must be used fresh, as quickly as possible. Raw living tissues may not be stored after any kind of preparation.- *A Cancer Therapy*, pg. 189
The following vegetables are very important (finely grated if necessary, or chopped, mixed or separate):

Knob Celery
Tomatoes
Escarole
Cauliflower
Romaine
Chives
Green Peppers
Apples and Carrots
Lettuce (all types)
Chicory
Watercress
Radishes
Scallions
Endives

Buttermilk Dressing*DAIRY, PG. 98
1 cup churned buttermilk (not cultured)
1/3 cup non-fat yogurt cheese
1/4 tsp. horseradish powder
2 tsp. honey
1 tsp. cider or wine vinegar
pinch dill, tarragon, or savory

Hand beat or buzz in blender until smooth. Leftover dressing may be kept in a tightly covered jar in the refrigerator for 48 hours.

Garlic & Onion Dressing (Salad Dressing 1)
2 tsp. Lemon Juice or Wine Vinegar
2 tsp. Water
1 tsp. Brown Sugar
a little Diced Onion
1 Clove Garlic
small amount of Permitted Herbs

Mix ingredients together, allow time for flavors to mingle, and serve on salad.

Herb Dressing (Salad Dressing 2)
1/3 cup Apple Cider Vinegar
1 tsp. Brown Sugar
2/3 cup Water

Mix these basic ingredients together and add some or all of the following (optional) and leave to infuse:

Tarragon, (pushed in stalk first)
Shallots or spring onions, chopped finely
2 cloves garlic, peeled and crushed with the back of a knife
1 fresh bay leaf

Orange Dill Vinaigrette
submitted by Richard Crowell
1/2 Cup Vinegar
3 Cloves Peeled Garlic
1 Cup Orange Juice
1/2 Cup Water
1 Green Onion
2 Tbsp. Honey
1/2 tsp. Dried Dill
1/4 Red Bell Pepper

Blend all ingredients in Osterizer. Makes 1 pint of zesty and sweet dressing.

Variation: Substitute juice of 1 Lime or Lemon for Orange Juice; increase Water. Substitute Sage or Thyme for Dill.

Spinach Dressing*DAIRY, PG. 98

1 Cup non-fat yogurt
2 Cups spinach chopped raw
or 1 Cup spinach, cooked
3 green onions chopped
1-2 tsp. vinegar
1/2 tsp. dill weed
pinch mace

Place in a blender & spin until smooth.

Yoguefort DressingDAIRY, PG. 98

3/4 Cup dry, unsalted
Cottage Cheese
1 Cup Yogurt
(or Churned Buttermilk)
1/4 Cup Vinegar or Lemon Juice
2 tsp. Honey
1 clove Garlic, crushed
1/4 tsp. Tarragon, Marjoram,
or Dill
1/4 Cup Chives
or Green Onions, chopped
2 Tbsp. Linseed Oil (optional)

Blend the first 5 ingredients in blender until smooth. Add herbs and chives. To thin mixture, add more yogurt. Chill before serving.

Summer Cole Slaw+DAIRY, PG. 98

1 Stalk Celery, finely chopped
1/4 Cup Minced Red Onion
1 1/2 Cups Shredded Cabbage
1/4 Cup Shredded Carrot
Pinch of Fresh Dill
2 Cups Non-Fat Yogurt

Combine all ingredients in bowl and toss well. Serve chilled.

Artichoke Salad

1 Purple Onion
1 Tomato
2 tbsp. Apple Cider Vinegar
1 Artichoke
1 Green Bell Pepper
2 Carrots
3 tbsp. Flax Seed Oil

Wash the artichokes well and boil in covered pot for 45 minutes to 1 hour. When ready, peel them until you can see the center. Remove the "chokes" with a spoon and discard. Cut the artichoke heart and other vegetables into bite size pieces. Combine and toss with vinegar and oil.

Bessarabian Nightmare+

2 tomatoes, sliced
1 small onion, sliced
1 red or green pepper (or both), sliced.
2-3 cloves of garlic, crushed
Permitted herbs to taste

Layer each ingredient in a glass pyrex baking dish. Bake at 350 degrees Fahrenheit until tender. Cool and add flax seed oil to taste when cool enough.

Celery Root (Knob) Salad

Remove loose roots from 2 Celery Knobs and scrub clean. Boil knobs in jacket about 1 hour, peel and slice

Add:

1 med. chopped Raw Onion
Scallions (green onion)

Toss with herb or Garlic-Onion salad dressing.

Cold Broccoli Salad*DAIRY, PG. 98

2 lbs. Broccoli

Cut broccoli into bite-sized pieces. Stew over a low flame in a heavy pan with a tight fitting cover until barely tender, about 25-30 minutes. Chill.

Add:

1 cup Cherry Tomatoes
1/2 cup Shallots
or Green Onions
1 cup Buttermilk Dressing
2-3 tsp. Chives
2-3 tsp. Parsley

Combine broccoli, tomatoes, and shallots in bowl. Mix in dressing. Serve on bed of Endive and garnish with Chives and Parsley

Eggplant Salad+

1 Eggplant

Bake eggplant for one hour at 350 degrees (180 degrees Celsius)
Let eggplant cool, then chop into bite - sized pieces.

Combine with:

1 small onion, chopped
1 tablespoon cider vinegar
Chopped parsley
2 sliced tomatoes
Flax oil

Fruity Winter SaladGSG DAIRY

1/2 white cabbage
2 med. carrots
2 red apples
1 oz. raisins
1 oz. dried figs
1 oz. dried apricots
10 Tbsp. non-fat yogurt
1 1/2 lemon
chopped parsley

Soak dried figs and apricots in bowl of

water overnight. The next day, empty water and add finely shredded cabbage, coarsely grated carrots and apples, and raisins. In a separate bowl, combine yogurt, lemon juice, and parsley. Combine contents of each bowl and toss together until well mixed. Serve chilled.

Italian Salad

Cauliflower
Broccoli
Celery
Tomatoes

Wash and cut up all vegetables, then toss with herb or garlic-onion salad dressing.

Peach Salad+

Mix together the following:

1 tomato, chopped
1 red pepper, chopped
1 green pepper, chopped
1 peach, chopped
½ cup green and red seedless grapes
A few mint leaves

Dress with lemon and garlic dressing: equal parts lemon juice and water. Add a little brown sugar (sucanat) and crushed garlic.

Potato Salad, Basic (1)

Boil potatoes until soft (1 hour) in jackets, peel and slice

Add:

Onions
Scallions
Celery
Green peppers
Herb or Garlic-Onion
Salad Dressing

Potato Salad, Fancy (2)

4 Potatoes
1 White Onion
1/4 Cup Celery
3 grated Carrots
Flax Seed Oil
2 Laurel Leaves
1 Purple Onion
Parsley
3 tbsp. Apple Cider Vinegar
1 Green Bell Pepper

Boil the potatoes in their jackets, with the laurel leaves on slow heat. Cut the vegetables and sauté with the apple cider vinegar (can use wok). No oil! Once the potatoes are cooked, peel, cut into small cubes and add the cooked vegetables. Add the flax seed oil after mixture is cooled.

Rice Salad+

Mix cooked, organic, brown rice (with bay leaf and a little rosemary) with plenty of chopped vegetables - tomatoes, celery, zucchini, radishes, fresh garden herbs and lemon and garlic dressing (see above).

Rose, borage and/or marigold petals look beautiful sprinkled over the salad. Add apricots which have been soaked in water and chopped (if desired).

Raw Grated Carrots & Apples

Grate by putting through grinder of Norwalk:

2 or 3 carrots
1 apple, peeled
Add 1/4 cup raisins
juice of 1/2 orange or lemon

Red And Green Salad*

Combine ingredients and serve with spinach dressing

1 head Romaine Lettuce
2 cup shredded Savoy or Green Cabbage
3 Green Onions
1 cup Sunflower Greens
2 Kohlrabi cut in shoe string strips or peeled broccoli stems
1 thinly sliced Yellow Crookneck Squash
1 pint Cherry Tomatoes or 1 large Sweet Red Pepper cut in strips

---

Sunchoke (Jerusalem Artichoke) Salad

Combine:

2 cup Sunchokes (cooked or raw)
1/2 cup Celery sliced diagonally
1/4 cup Green Peppers
1/2 cup Salad Dressing

Tomato and Pepper Salad+

1 Green pepper, cut into thin rings
2 Tomatoes, firm but ripe, sliced or chopped

Dress with lemon juice and crushed garlic, fresh herbs and chopped celery leaves. Add flax oil to taste.

Beet Salad

Boil Beets in Water for 1 hour. Peel and cut tips off, slice thin. Add Chopped Onions and either Herb or Garlic-Onion salad dressing.

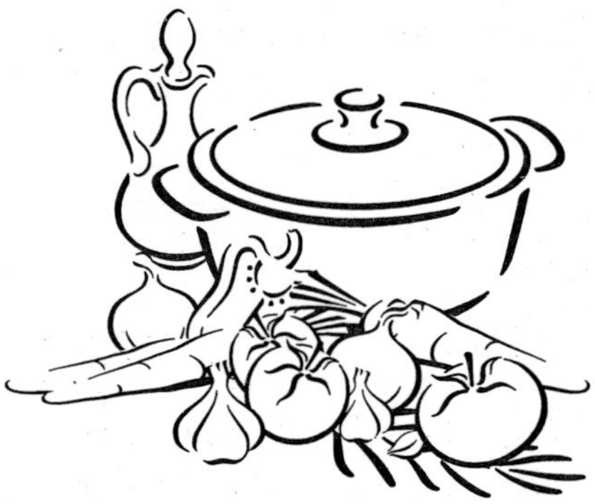

Cooked Vegetable Dishes

Preparation Of Vegetables:
All vegetables must be cooked slowly, over low flame, with little or no addition of water. The slow cooking process is very important, in order to preserve the natural flavor of the vegetables and keep them easily digestible. All vegetables should be "done" or tender. Valuable components are lost in fast cooking by excessive heat, because the cells burst, the minerals go out of their colloidal composition and become more difficult to be absorbed. A stainless steel "flame tamer" may be used to prevent burning. A little of the "Special Soup" may also be used, or tomatoes, apple slices, or chopped onion may be placed at the bottom of the pan to give up more fluid. In some cases this also improves the flavor. Only spinach water is too bitter, contains too much oxalic acid and must be discarded. Tomatoes, leeks, zucchini and onions should be stewed in their own juices, as they contain an abundance of fluid by themselves. Red beets should be cooked like potatoes, in their peel, in water. All vegetables must be carefully washed and cleaned. Peeling or scraping is forbidden, because important mineral salts and vitamins are deposited directly under the skin. The pot (not aluminum) must close tightly, to prevent escape of steam. Don't use pressure cooking pots. Lids must be heavy and fit well into the pots. Cooked foods (soup and fruit) may be kept in the refrigerator for 48 hours.

Baked vegetables should be slow cooked in a "low" oven (180-190 degrees, use oven thermometer) for 2 to 2 and 1/2 hours, in a covered casserole with a tightly fitting lid. This method of baking is virtually waterless. Use onions, tomatoes, or sprinkle vegetables with lemon to add moisture when necessary.

Stewed vegetables are cooked in a heavy pot with tightly fitting lid on top of the stove over a low flame, slowly with little or no added liquid.

Simmered vegetables are cooked on the top of the stove over a low flame in a tightly covered pan with a small amount of liquid. The temperature is kept just at the boiling point.

Boiled vegetables (like corn and artichokes) are cooked on the top of the stove in a heavy pot with a tightly fitting lid. Place 1 inch of cold water in the bottom of the pot, add the washed vegetables (do not peel or scrape), cover. Cook over medium heat, slowly bringing the liquid to a boil (bubbles breaking on the surface and steam given off). Lower the flame as much as possible, keeping the liquid boiling. Note: Bring liquids to a boil only if the recipe specifically calls for it.

"Tightly Fitting Lids": saucepans must be tightly covered to prevent steam from escaping. Covers must be heavy and close fitting. You may have to place wax paper under the lid to aid the seal.

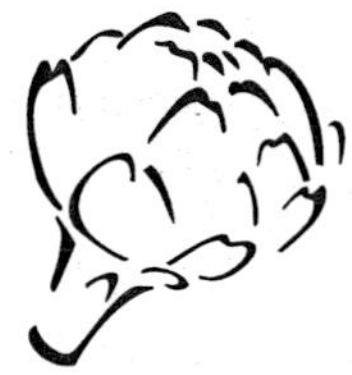

Artichokes
Cut ends and rinse in the center
Bring 2 inches of water to a boil
Add Artichokes. Lower temperature, cover and simmer for approximately 1 hour. Serve with salad dressing on the side as a dip.

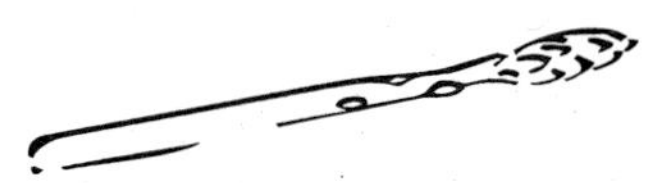

Asparagus
Bake in covered casserole with a small amount of soup stock or lemon juice in low oven 1 hour or simmer with 1/2" soup stock for 30 minutes or until tender.

Beautiful Borscht+

1 onion
3 garlic cloves
1 cup Special Soup
6 small beets with tops
1 large potato
1 carrot
4 red cabbage leaves
2 bay leaves
3 cups water
2 tomatoes

Run all the vegetables through your grinder and add the water and bay leaves. Cook for 30 minutes on low heat. Serve with a dab of non-fat yogurt.

Beets
Bake or boil beets in their jackets.

Glazed Beets*

(serves 6-8)

9 Large Beets

Scrub 9 beets and boil in 1" water until tender, approx. 1 to 1 1/2 hours. Peel in cold water. Slice or cut into bit sized pieces.

Glaze for Beets

Combine:

2/3 cup fresh orange juice
1 tsp. cornstarch
1 1/2 tsp. cider vinegar
1 tsp. honey
or crude brown sugar

Cook over low flame until thick. Add Beets and mix well. **Variation**: Use 1/2 cup apple juice and 3 tsp. lemon juice in place of orange juice.

Beets, Cooked & "Creamed"DAIRY

3 cooked beets
6 Tbsp. non-fat yogurt
1 Tbsp. fresh snipped chives
2 Tbsp. finely chopped onion
finely chopped parsley

Put cooked, chopped beets into a saucepan with the yogurt, chives and onion and heat gently. Put into serving dish and sprinkle with chopped parsley.

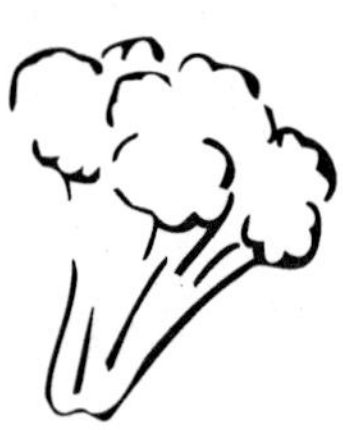

Broccoli

Bake in a covered casserole in low oven with onions or a small amount of soup stock for 1-2 hours. Serve with tomato sauce.

Broccoli & HerbsMZ

2 bunches of broccoli
4-6 cloves of garlic
1/2 onion, sliced
1/4 tsp. dill
1/4 Cup Special Soup broth

Wash broccoli and peal stems. Put garlic and onion in one pot and cook until onion becomes translucent. Add cut broccoli crowns and stems, dill and broth. Cook on low heat until broccoli is tender.

Festive Broccoli* (or Festive Green Beans)

*1 large bunch broccoli**
1 clove garlic, minced
1 small onion, diced
1 medium sweet red or yellow bell pepper, cut in strips
2 tsp. lemon juice (optional)
1/4 tsp. dried or 1 tsp.
fresh dillweed

* This recipe works well with green beans as well. Replace broccoli with;

3 1/2 cups sliced beans.

Select dark green bunch of broccoli with no yellowing. Wash well and cut into spears, peeling tougher stalks at base. Place onion, and garlic in pot. Cover and stew on low flame for 45 min. or until tender. Add pepper strips for last 20-25 minutes of cooking. Add lemon just before serving - will discolor broccoli if added during cooking. Sprinkle vegetables with dill and serve.

Cauliflower

Wash and break into sections. 2-3 tomatoes, sliced and cut into chunks. Stew for approximately 45 minutes (or until tender) on low heat.

Cauliflower and Carrot Sauce

1 small Cauliflower
3 carrots
Flax Seed Oil

Separate the Cauliflowerets and place in a baking dish with a little water and cook until soft at 250 degrees. When ready, drain off the water. At the same time, simmer the carrots on low heat with enough water until they are soft. Blend Carrots in blender with the oil. Pour sauce over the cooked Cauliflower, and place in warm oven (turned off) for 5-10 minutes, before serving.

Carrots and Honey

Wash Carrots, cut off ends, and slice. Do not peel or scrape. Stew in a small amount of soup stock for 45 minutes or until tender. Last 5-10 min.

add:

1/2 tsp. Honey for slight flavoring

Chard Rolls, StuffedMZ

1 bunch of chard
6 medium potatoes
4 carrots
1/2 onion, sliced
3 large cloves of garlic, minced

Cook onions and potatoes separately. In another pot, cook carrots and garlic. When done, puree each potfull separately, then mix together. Put chard leaves in very hot water, assuring not to overcook. Spread each leaf and remove tough center stem. Then place puree in center of leaf and roll tightly. Display on tray and serve with "ketchup" (see recipe, pg. 92).

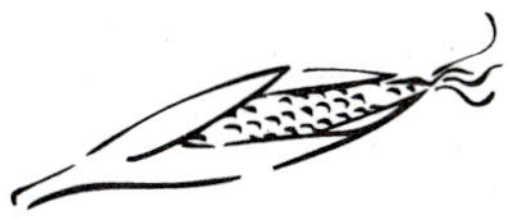

Corn

Corn may be baked in the husk wrapped in foil. Bake in low oven for 1 hour or place in boiling water for approximately 7 minutes

---

Corn with Mixed Vegetables

3 stalks of Celery
2 Carrots
2 ears of Corn
2 Zucchini Squash

Wash the corn well and husk it. Cut the kernels off. Slice the other vegetables into smaller pieces. Put the corn in a baking dish and add the vegetables. Bake in the oven at 200 degrees for 1 hour.

Creamed Corn

3 ears of Corn
1 Green Bell Pepper

Husk corn and cut off the kernels. Put kernels from 2 ears in a blender and blend. Add the kernels from the third ear to the blended corn. Place in a baking dish and on the top place sliced green pepper. Bake in the oven 1 1/2 hours at 200-250 degrees.

Corn With Orange Juice

2 ears of Corn
1 glass of Orange Juice

Wash the corn well, husk, and cut off the kernels. Put this in a baking dish with a lid and bake in the oven at 250 degrees until done. Pour the corn juice off, and add the orange juice. Let set 5-10 minutes before serving.

Dilly Beans *

3 cups Green Beans
1/3 cup Onion sliced in half rings
1/2 tsp. Dill Weed
2 tsp. Lemon Juice
Green Or White Cabbage

Combine in pan:

1/2 Cabbage, shredded thinly
pinch marjoram
3-4 tsp. Apple Cider Vinegar
1 large Tomato
Chopped Sage
1 Onion, diced

Combine and bake in low oven in a covered casserole until tender. Stew approximately 1 hour, until tender. Do not add water

---

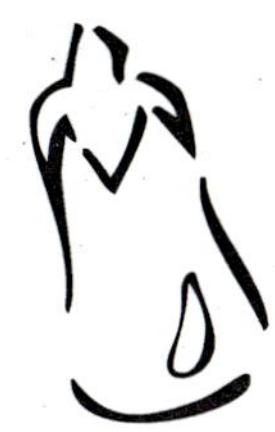

Eggplant, Baked

Put some soup stock in bottom of large covered baking dish

Add in layers:

1 chopped Onion
1 Eggplant, sliced
2 Tomatoes, sliced and skinned

Cover and bake In low oven for 2 hours.

Eggplant, Stewed

Combine in stew pot:

1 eggplant, cut into cubes
2 onions, chopped
3 tomatoes (peeled and chopped)

Stew approximately 30 minutes (until tender). Do not add water.

Eggplant Roulades DAIRY, PG. 98 with Red Pepper Sauce

The Sauce:

1 red pepper, quartered & de-seeded
1 onion, finely chopped
2 tomatoes, chopped
1 clove garlic, crushed
6 Tbsp. water

The Roulade:

2 eggplants
1 pot of cottage cheese (unsalted, non-fat)
2 tomatoes, skinned and chopped
herbs (such as parsley or coriander)

To make the sauce, cook the pepper, onion, tomatoes and garlic in the water, and simmer for 20 minutes. Put through the food processor or blender. For the roulade, cut the eggplants lengthways into 1/4 slices. Put in an oven-proof dish and cook a little in the oven to soften them. In the meantime, mix together the cottage cheese and herbs and prepare the tomatoes. Then spread a little cottage cheese over each partially cooked piece of eggplant, scatter with tomatoes and roll up. Place back into the oven-proof dish and cook for 15-20 minutes. Serve hot, garnished with the pepper sauce.

Fennel Treat+

1 bulb of fennel
1 large tomato cut into ¼ inch slices
2-3 cloves garlic, peeled, sliced thin

Cut stalks and leaves off fennel. Slice bulb in half lengthwise so you have two flat halves. Rinse halves under running water to remove sand and put them in a baking dish with cut side up. Cover halves with tomato slices and place garlic slices on top of tomatoes. Cover dish and bake at 250 degrees for 1-2 hours. Serve with a baked potato and a salad of grated carrots on a bed of pretty greens.

Green Chard Rolls

4 leaves of Green Chard
2 Carrots
1/4 head Broccoli
2 cloves Garlic
1/2 Cup Rice, uncooked
1/4 head Cauliflower
2 small Zucchini Squash
1 ear of Corn (cut kernels off)
1 1/2 Tomatoes

Wash the vegetables well. Put the chard leaves in hot water long enough to wilt them so they will bend. Cut the other vegetables into small pieces, and put them in a pan with a little bit of water to boil on low heat. When cooked, drain the water off. Make a sauce in the blender with the tomatoes and garlic, and pour this sauce on top of the vegetables and raw rice. Place some of the vegetables-rice mixture in the center of each leaf and roll them up. Put these in a baking dish with a lid and bake in the oven for 1 to 1 1/2 hours at 250 degrees.

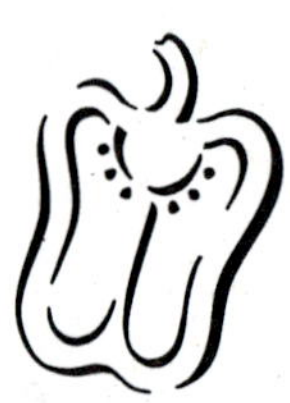

Green Peppers

2-4 sliced green peppers
2-4 sliced onions

Stew in tightly covered pot approximately 30 min. (add no water)

Lima Beans And Zucchini

1 large Onion
1 clove Garlic
1/2 Cup Soup Stock
1 Cup fresh Lima Beans
3 Cups Zucchini
4 med. Tomatoes
1/2 tsp. Cornstarch
4 sprigs fresh Parsley
dash Thyme and Sage
or pinch dried Parsley

Mix all ingredients except herbs. Simmer about 15 minutes (until tender) Thicken with cornstarch mixed with a little water. Just before serving add herbs.

Onions and Raisins

1 Onion, peeled and chopped
1/4 cup Raisins

Stew in tightly covered pot approximately 30 minutes.

Onions, Cheese MarinatedDAIRY, PG. 98

2 Tbsp. lemon juice
3 oz. pot cheese (unsalted, non-fat)
1/2 tsp. brown sugar
2 Cups onions, sliced thick

Stuffed Pepper+DAIRY, PG. 98

1 large green or red pepper
4 oz. pot cheese
¼ onion
1 zucchini
1 small carrot
3 tomatoes
1 small turnip
1 clove garlic
1 tablespoon fresh mixed herbs
4 oz. Hippocrates soup

Put the pepper in a saucepan with a little water and cook over low heat (covered) until tender. Remove from the pan and leave the pepper upside down to drain and cool.

Finely chop the onion, zucchini, carrot, herbs, tomatoes, turnip and garlic. Place in a small saucepan with the soup and simmer over low heat for 45 minutes to an hour.

Core the pepper with a sharp knife, removing all seeds.

Mix the pot cheese with the cooked vegetables and fill the pepper using a small spoon.

Stand the pepper in a suitable baking dish and bake for 40 minutes at 350 degrees.

Serve with French Tomato Sauce, baked potato and a green vegetable.

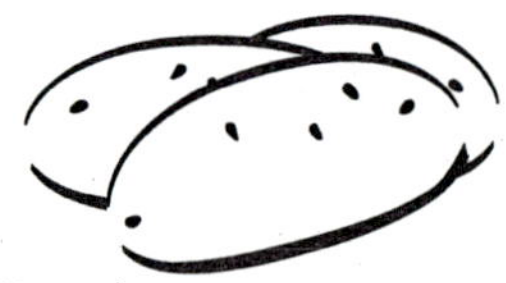

Potatoes

Potatoes are most often boiled slowly in a covered pot over medium-low heat approximately 1 hour, until tender.

Baked Potatoes

Baked potatoes should be thoroughly washed, not scraped or peeled. Bake in a low oven for 2-2 and 1/2 hours or bake 50 minutes to 1 hour at 350 degrees.

Mashed Potatoes

Peel and cube potatoes. Place in pan with one small onion and enough water to bring to a boil and simmer until done. When done, there should be no water left. Mash with enough non-fat yogurt to make smooth.

Mashed Potatoes and Chard

Take one bunch of chard, green or red, wash and shred and put in pan. Add small amount (4-5 Tbsp.) of water or soup stock, and start to boil. when boiling, turn down to simmer. Meantime, peel 3 large or four medium/large potatoes; cube and place on top of the chard. Let simmer until potatoes are soft and done.

Remove water if any remains, and add approximately 6-8 oz. of non-fat yogurt. Mash all together. Add a little more yogurt if the mixture is too dry. The same recipe can be used with kale. When using kale, remove central stems, by stripping them before shredding into pan.

Parsley Potatoes

Boil several potatoes in their skins until done. Remove the peel and roll in some chopped parsley after slightly brushing with flaxseed oil.

Potato Puffs

(marginal food, to be eaten only rarely)

Take a baking potato and cut it into thin (1/2") slices. Place the slices on the oven rack and, without any addition, bake at HIGH heat (425 F) to puff, turn over and lower heat to 325° F (with oven door cracked). Bake for another 20 minutes. The slices puff up and become crisp and tasty, almost like fried potatoes. Done when shiny brown on both sides.

Scalloped Potatoes

Take a glass baking dish and place one whole chopped onion in bottom. Slice potatoes and place one layer on top of the onion. Then place a layer of sliced tomato on top, another layer of sliced or chopped onion. Sprinkle with a dash of marjoram and/or thyme and bake in a low oven 1-2 hours or until done.

Potatoes and Carrots, Westphalian Style

6-8 small Carrots, sliced
or 4-5 large Carrots, sliced
3 medium potatoes
or 2 large Potatoes
1 large onion
3-4 Tbsp. Soup stock

Wash and slice carrots into pan. Peel and slice potatoes and chop onion. Add all together in pan with soup stock. Let simmer until done, adding a bit more Soup Stock if necessary. When done, no water should remain in pan.

Red Cabbage

Combine in pan:

1/2 Cabbage, shredded
3 tsp. Vinegar
3 large Chopped Onions
2 Bay Leaves
a little Soup Stock

Stew over low heat approximately 1/2 hour.

Last half hour add:

3 Apples, peeled and grated
1 tsp. Raw Sugar

Spinach

After cutting off roots wash 3-4 times. Put in large, tightly covered pot which has a layer of onions on the bottom of the pan. Do not add water. Stew over a low flame until spinach wilts. Pour off excess juice Serve chopped with slice of lemon

Stuffed Holiday Squash*

1 Lrg. Kabocha squash
(about 4 1/2 lbs.)
3/4 Cup raw brown rice
1/4 Cup raw wild rice, rye or wheat berries, or more brown rice
2 1/2 cups vegetable stock
or purified water
1 Cup onion, diced
3 cloves garlic, minced
1 1/2 cup fresh peas, shelled,
or sprouted lentils
3/4 Cup celery, diced
3/4 Cup yellow or red bell pepper, diced
1/2 Cup unsulphured raisins
or prunes (pit prunes and chop)
1 tsp. each sage and savory
2 tsp. thyme
1/3 Cup fresh parsley,
finely chopped
1/4 Cup fresh orange juice

* I love the texture and taste of this Japanese squash - it's very meaty and sweet, but you could use pumpkin, turban or acorn squash (cut latter in half and seed). You may also use 2 or 3 smaller sized squashes rather than a large one. This makes a very attractive presentation, especially if the squash are of different sizes.

Cook rice and wild rice together in vegetable stock for 45 minutes or until rice is done. Using stock to cook the grain adds both nutrition and flavor. Just save your vegetable trimmings, carrots, parsnips, chard stems or greens, celery, celery root, onion all work well. Avoid cabbage family veggies as they impart a strong flavor. Cover with pure water and simmer until done. Use in soups, to make sauces or what have you.

Carefully cut the top off of the squash as you would when carving a pumpkin. Remove seeds. Place squash face down on baking pan together with the squash lid and prebake for 25 to 30 minutes in a 350 degree oven. Take care not to over cook - a mushy squash cannot be stuffed.

Place onion and garlic, peas and celery in a pot and cook on low for 20 minutes to barely tenderize. Add diced pepper, raisins, herbs, citrus juice, and cooked rice, mixing well. Fill squash with stuffing, packing it down. Return to oven and bake 25 to 30 minutes, or until squash is tender, but still firm. If there is extra filling, bake in a covered casserole with a tablespoon of stock or juice, or fill a bell pepper or two and do the same.

To serve, arrange a platter with fresh

kale or other leafy greens. Place squash in center of platter and artistically prop squash fid up against squash. Spoon out each helping, making sure to get some of the delicious squash meat. Alternatively, if squash is cooled a bit before serving, it may be sliced in wedges. Ladle Parsley Yogurt Sauce (see recipe below) over each portion, if dairy is allowed, otherwise a squeeze of orange juice adds a bit of zing. Enjoy!

Stuffed Squash*

3-4 Acorn Squash
1/2 Cup Onion, diced
1/2 Cup Celery, diced
1/2 Cup Carrot, diced
1 1/4 Cup cooked Brown Rice
1/2 Cup Lentils, sprouted
1/4 Cup Raisins or chopped prunes, soaked & drained
3 tsp. fresh parsley, minced
1/2 tsp. rubbed sage
1/2 tsp. thyme
*1 large clove garlic, crushed***

Slice squash lengthwise and remove seeds. Combine remaining ingredients, fill squash halves. Cover and bake at 300 - 325 degrees F., for 1 1/2 hours, or until squash is tender. Delicious with Apricot Sauce or Golden Gravy (see Sauces & Dips).
***Try using 6-8 whole cloves garlic for a delicious mild flavor. Crushing releases the strong aromatic oils, whereas using garlic uncut imparts a very mild flavor.*

Stir Steam Snow Peas Medley

submitted by Richard Crowell

1 Pound Snow Peas
1 Bunch Bok Choy
1 Medium Zucchini
1 Medium Crookneck Yellow Squash
1 Small Red Onion
1 Carrot
1 Leek
1 Cup Orange Juice
1 Tbsp. Honey
1 Tbsp. Vinegar
1 tsp. Allspice

Clean all vegetables, removing stem from snow peas, slicing white stalk and green leaf of bok choy into strips, slicing yellow squash lengthwise and then into half circles. You can make attractive planks out of the zucchini by trimming off each end, and then cutting in half, then half again. Stand each barrel of squash on end and slice down into 1/8" planks. Dice red onion, then slice carrots oriental style as thin as possible at a 45 degree angle into ovals. Slice leek in similar fashion across stalk into ovals. Put orange juice, honey, allspice, and vinegar into a blender, then pour into a suitable-sized steam pot. Cover with all the vegetables and simmer 15-20 minutes until tender. Very succulent!

String Beans

1 lb. Green Beans (cut tips, wash and cut into any size piece desired)
Add:
1 med. Onion, chopped
some Soup Stock (just enough to keep beans moist)
Stew approximately 50 minutes (until tender)

Sweet Potato

Cut off tips and wash
Perforate with knife to let steam escape place in casserole (covered for soft skin, uncovered for crisp skin) bake in low oven for 2 to 2 and 1/2 hours.

Tomatoes, Grilled

Slice tomatoes in half
Put in pan, sliced side up, cover each half with chopped onions bake in low oven 1 hour. Save juice to put into soup

---

Green Tomato Mincemeat

1 qt. Green Tomatoes
2 oz. Golden Raisins
1/2 cup Brown Sugar
1/4 cup Water
2 oz. Seeded Raisins
1/4 tsp. Cloves
1/4 cup Wine Vinegar
1 pt. tart Apples

Put tomatoes through coarse chopper. Combine all ingredients except apples. Heat to tender about 30 min. stirring. Add chopped apples and cook until thick.

Tomatoes Stuffed with Mixed Vegetables

4 Tomatoes

Vegetables: as much of as many kinds as desired

2 Tomatoes
6 Garlic Cloves

Wash tomatoes well. Hollow out the four tomatoes. Cut the vegetables into small pieces and boil in a little water for half an hour. Put cooked vegetables in the tomatoes and place them in a baking dish without the lid. In the blender, blend the two tomatoes and garlic. Spread sauce on top of each tomato. Preheat oven for ten minutes. Turn it off. Put tomatoes in for another ten minutes.

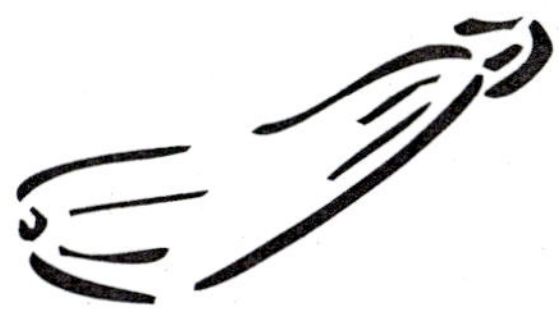

Zucchini

Combine:

sliced Zucchini
raw chopped Onion
chopped Tomatoes
touch of Soup Stock

Stew for 20 minutes or cut squash into small pieces and place in a baking dish. In the blender blend the tomatoes, onion, and 4 garlic cloves. Pour sauce over squash and bake 1 & 1/2 hours at 200-250 degrees.

Zucchini And Rice

1/2 lb. organic Brown Rice
1 Carrot
1 Zucchini
2 Garlic Cloves

Wash the rice and vegetables well. Put rice in a baking dish and add chopped up parsley, carrot, celery, and zucchini squash. At the same time blend tomato and garlic in the blender and spread on top of the rice and vegetables. Bake in the oven for 1 & 1/2 hours at 250 degrees.

Zucchini and Tomatoes+

6 small zucchini, sliced
1 medium or large onion, chopped
2-3 tomatoes, chopped
Garlic and herbs to taste (thyme, mace, marjoram)

Saute onion, tomatoes and seasonings in a little water. Add zucchini when half done, and simmer. Serve as a vegetable or potato topping.

Spaghetti With Beetballs *

Wash one medium spaghetti squash and cut in half. Scoop out seeds and place cut side down on baking sheet. Bake in low oven for 2 hours or until tender. OR place cut side up in a large covered pot with 1" water and steam over low flame for 1 hour or until done.

Note: *Spaghetti squash is a yellow hard winter squash developed by a Japanese farmer some 30 years ago. When cooked, it comes out in strands like spaghetti. It is now widely available especially in organic growers' circles.*

Sauce

2 lb. ripe Tomatoes (6-8 large)
3-5 cloves Garlic, minced
1 med. Onion, diced fine
1 Green Pepper, diced
2 stalks Celery, diced
or 1 sm. Fennel Bulb, diced
2 sm. Zucchini, sliced
or 1 cup Eggplant, cubed
4 tsp. fresh Parsley, minced
*pinch each Rosemary, Thyme, Sage & Marjoram**
1/2 tsp. Fennel Seeds

Cook whole tomatoes over a low flame for 30-35 min. or until tender. To ensure a thick, rich sauce, pour off the extra juice drawn from the tomatoes during cooking.** Put drained tomatoes through food mill or sieve to remove skins and seeds. Pour sauce back into pot and add remaining veggies and seasonings. Cover and stew over low flame for 1 hr. or until veggies are done to your liking. For a little extra bite add a dash or two of wine vinegar with a tsp. of honey.

*Basil and oregano, both favorite Italian seasonings, are not allowed on Gerson Therapy due to the aromatic oils they contain.

**Please be sure to keep extra tomato liquid for soup or gravy, or better still, drink as a hot broth immediately. It's delicious.

Beet Balls

2 tsp. Parsley, minced
1 sm. Onion, minced
1 med. Beet, grated
3-4 med. Carrots, grated
OR 1 cup Eggplant, ground
1/2 cup Essene Rye Bread or Saltless, Fatless Rye
*1 1/2 cup 2 day old Lentils, germinated**
1 sm. bunch Endive, Spinach or young Chard, finely chopped
2-3 cloves Garlic, minced

Put lentils and eggplant (if used) through food grinder or Norwalk Juicer using grid #2. Mix with bread crumbs and remaining veggies. Mix well. Form into 2" balls and place on baking sheet well sprinkled with oat or rye meal to prevent sticking. Cover and bake in low oven for 1 hour. Uncover and bake 1 hour more.

Arrange cooked spaghetti squash on a plate with one or two beet balls, cover with sauce and enjoy!

*Cover lentils with distilled water and allow to soak (germinate) overnight. Drain.

Variations

Use 3 large white or 3 med. sweet potatoes in place of ground lentils. Boil until tender, then put through food mill or grinder with skins. Proceed as with above. Replace bread crumbs with 1/2 cup cooked brown rice or 1/3 cup oat flakes ground in Norwalk.

Veggie Loaf*

Grind in Norwalk or food grinder:

*2 Cup lentils, germinated**
1/4 Cup fresh parsley
1 1/2 Cup eggplant, diced or Parsnips or Yams

Add:

1 Cup Onions diced fine
3/4 Cup Beets, grated
3/4 Cup Carrots grated
1 Cup Celery diced fine
3 cloves Garlic, minced
1 1/2 Cups cooked Brown Rice
pinch Thyme
pinch Rubbed Sage
pinch Tarragon
1 tsp. Lemon Juice

Bake in covered pan in low oven for approximately 2 hours. Uncover and baste with Golden Sauce or Tomato sauce. Bake another 30 minutes to 1 hour. Serve with extra sauce.

Veggie Stroganoff* DAIRY, PG. 98

1 Cup onion, diced
1 Cup eggplant, diced
1-1/2 Cups cauliflowerets or cabbage
1-1/2 Cups sliced carrots or tomatoes
1 Cup broccoli or green pepper
1 Cup celery or zucchini, sliced

Stew vegetables for 1-1/2 hours until tender (you may want to add soft veggies like tomatoes and zucchini last). Set aside and let cool to 140 degrees while making sauce as follows:

3 tbsp. wine or cider vinegar
1 tsp. dillweed
2 Cup yogurt
1 Cup cottage cheese (non-fat, saltless) green onions or parsley for garnish

Blend sauce until smooth. Mix with warm veggies. Serve over a bed of baked spaghetti squash or cooked brown rice. Garnish with chopped green onions or parsley.

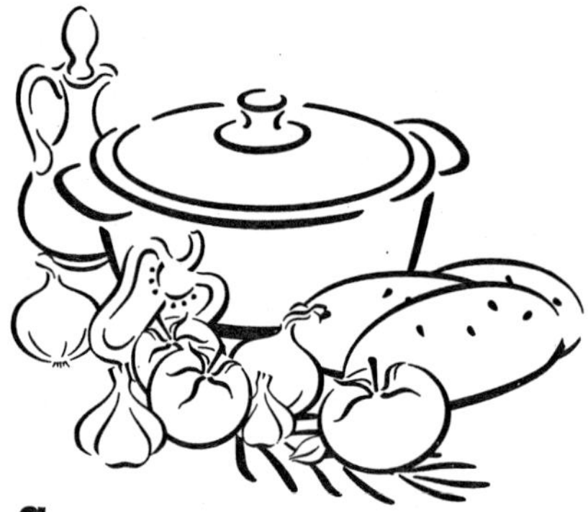

Soups

Potato Soup

1 large Onion
1/2 small Celery Knob
Parsley
2 large Potatoes
1 Leek
2 stalks Celery
2 quarts Water

Clean and dice all vegetables. Place in covered saucepan with water. Bring to boil. Lower heat. Cover. Simmer 2-3 hours. Mash through food mill.

Special Soup

(See page 80 for recipe)

Tomato Soup with Lemon & Garlic

2 to 3 large Tomatoes
1 clove Garlic
1 Bay Leaf
juice of 1/2 Lemon
2 Onions
1 tsp. Oats Flakes
1 tsp. Brown Sugar
1/2 cup Soup Stock (see above)

Dice all vegetables. Place vegetables-soup stock-sugar and lemon in covered saucepan and cook for 1 hour. Mash through food mill. Replace in saucepan. Add oat flakes and cook 5 more minutes.

Tomato and Mint Soup GSG

2 lbs. tomatoes (roma preferrably)
5 green onions (scallions)
2 small cooking apples
5 Tbsp. cider vinegar
1 tsp. brown sugar
2 large lemons
6-8 sprigs fresh mint
200 g. (6-8 oz.) nonfat yogurt (optional) DAIRY, PG. 98

Chop tomatoes, slice spring onions, core and slice apple. Put these into a saucepan with the cider vinegar and sugar. Bring to a boil and simmer gently for 30 minutes. Put through food mill.

Either leave to cool, adding last ingredients later, or add the lemon juice and beat in the yogurt (if opted) immediately. Just before serving, add the chopped mint, leaving some scattered over the top of the soup for decoration.

Makes four generous, or six small servings.

Tomato Soup with Potato & Onion

2 large Tomatoes
1 medium Onion
1 tsp. Brown Sugar
2 medium Potatoes
1 tsp. Wine Vinegar
small piece of Bay Leaf

Wash and dice all vegetables. Place all ingredients except sugar in covered saucepan with water to cover. Cook over low flame for 1 hour. Mash through food mill and add sugar to taste.

Sauces & Dips

Apricot Sauce

1/4 cup dried Apricots, unsulphured
1 cup pure Water, heated
1/2 cup fresh Apple
or Orange Juice

Wash and drain apricots. Combine with water and soak for several hours. Add juice and stew over low flame until apricots are very tender, about 1 1/2 hours. Puree sauce in blender or by putting through Foley Food Mill or Norwalk.

Baba Ghanoush

1 large eggplant
2 cloves garlic
1 tsp lemon juice
1 tablespoon chopped parsley
Lemon wedges

Bake eggplant for one hour and when cool enough, peel and drain off excess liquid, squeezing gently. Blend with garlic until fairly smooth, add lemon juice and parsley. Mix well. Serve with raw dipping vegetables such as celery, carrots, cauliflower, peppers.

Golden Gravy

1 sm. Potato, quartered
4 Carrots, sliced
2 tsp. Cider Vinegar or Lemon Juice
1 cup Soup Stock or Water
1 sm. Onion, diced
1/4 tsp. Dill, Marjoram or Thyme
1 tsp. Parsley, minced

Combine ingredients and stew over low flame for 1 1/2 to 2 hours or until tender. Remove potato skins and puree.

Golden Sauce

Combine in a covered casserole:

1 small sweet potato or yam quartered
2-3 carrots coarsely chopped
1 small onion, diced
1/2 cup soup stock
1/2 cup tangerine or orange juice
pinch thyme and rosemary

Bake in low oven until tender (approx. 2 hours) Put through Foley food mill or spin in blender adding more juice to achieve desired consistency. Add 2 tsp. parsley and serve.

Ketchup/Catsup

3 tomatoes
1/2 head of garlic
1/2 onion
1/16 Cup (1/2 oz.) vinegar
1/4 tsp. dill
1/2 Cup Sucanat (organic brown sugar)

Place all ingredients in pan and bring to a boil. Cook until tender and put through food mill or liquefier until smooth.

Parsley Yogurt Sauce DAIRY, PG. 98

1/2 Cup minced onion
1 tsp. fresh grated horseradish
or 1/2 tsp. dried horseradish (opt.)
1 Cup nonfat yogurt
1 Tbsp. lemon or lime juice
1 tsp. maple syrup or honey
1/4 Cup minced parsley

Cook onions over low heat until tender and translucent. Remove from heat and let cool slightly. Blend onions with horseradish, yogurt, citrus juice and sweetener in blender until smooth. Stir in parsley.

Marjoram

Plum Sauce

1/2 lb. plums
1/2 tsp. lemon juice
1 slice toast diced
1 tsp. brown sugar
2 tsp. bread crumbs

Wash plums. Remove pits and place in saucepan with water to half cover. Cook 15 minutes and strain through food mill. Add sugar, bread crumbs, lemon juice. Replace in saucepan. Cook 3 minutes longer. Serve over toast if desired.

Tomato Salsa

1 medium tomato, finely chopped
Green onions or 1 medium red onion
2 Tbsp. fresh coriander
leaves (cilantro), chopped
3 Tbsp. lemon juice

Combine ingredients (don't overdo the lemon juice), cover and chill. Best eaten fresh but can be kept for up to 2 days in the refrigerator.

Tomato Sauce, No Wait

(This sauce is raw)

1 lb. Roma Tomatoes,
cut into pieces
3-4 cloves of Garlic
3 sprigs of Parsley Herbs
1 tsp. Linseed Oil

Place linseed oil in blender and start. Begin adding pieces of tomato and other ingredients a little bit at a time. Allow to whip for a minute or so until all ingredients are mixed. Yields about 2-3 cup of sauce.

Tomato Sauce

Combine in large pan:

4-6 large tomatoes
4-5 large Onions, peeled and sliced
1 large, or 2 medium Potatoes with

skins, diced
2-3 cloves Garlic
pinch Marjoram
pinch Thyme

Stew and let simmer for 1 hour and pass through Foley food mill. One can also add a little celery or green pepper for taste.

Tomato Sauce, French

Makes 1.25 pints

1 onion
½ stick celery
½ small carrot
1 ¼ pounds tomatoes
A few sprigs of flat leaf parsley
1 clove garlic
1 bay leaf

Cook chopped onion, carrot, celery tomatoes, parsley, garlic and bay leaf. Puree and serve hot or cold.

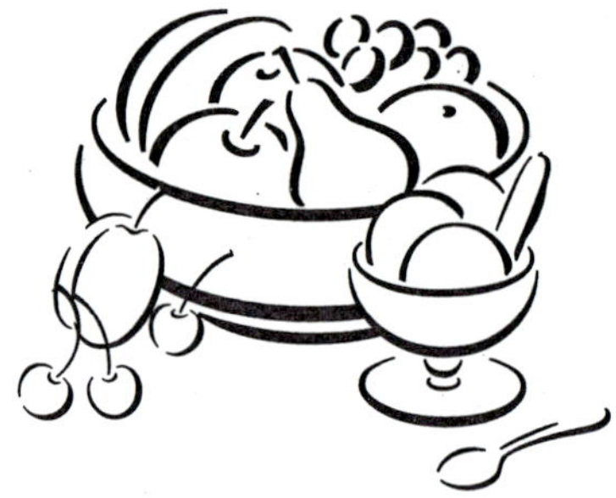

Fruits & Desserts

Fruits

Most fresh fruits can be eaten when ripe unpeeled. Of course fruits like oranges and bananas should be peeled. Always wash fresh fruit.

Dried fruits should be washed in clean, lukewarm, distilled water and soaked over night in water (little more than to cover). Use the same water and cook in covered saucepan until tender. Dried fruits must be unsulfured.

The following fruit recipes are taken from Dr. Gerson's personal files.

Desserts

Desserts should never replace the meals or juices of the therapy. At the risk of sounding like your mother, "Clean your plate before dessert, dear!" Do not eat or use as ingredients in desserts: ice-cream, fat, white flour, baking soda, candy, chocolate, cream, or salt. Have fun!

Sugar

Use only brown (Sucanator raw sugar, light honey, maple syrup or unsulfured molasses.

Syrup

Boil 1 lb. brown sugar in 1 quart of water and 1 cup apple juice until dissolved. Keep in covered jar.

Apples, Baked

2 medium Apples
1 tsp. Raisins
6 tsp. Water

Wash, core and cut apples in half. Place with raisins in pan or baking dish in oven for about 15 minutes until done then broil under flame until golden brown about 5 minutes. Apple halves should stay whole. Honey may be added to raisins - to taste.

Apple and Banana

1/2 cup Apple Sauce
1/2 raw Sliced Banana
juice of 1/2 Lemon

Serve raw or place applesauce and banana in covered saucepan and heat slowly. Serve with lemon juice.

Apple Cake with Maple Yogurt DAIRY, PG. 98

1 1/2 lbs. cooking apples
1 lemon
1 oz. rolled oats
1 oz. oatmeal
2 oz. sultanas or raisins
4 oz. brown sugar
4 oz. wholewheat flour
1 tsp. potassium baking powder
1/2 Cup fresh apple juice
yogurt
maple syrup

Put peeled and chopped apples into a large bowl and sprinkle with lemon juice. Combine rolled oats, oatmeal, raisins, sugar, flour and baking powder and mix well. Stir this mixture into the apples. Pour mixture into cake pan and bake at 350 degrees F for 20-35 minutes or until lightly browned on top. Serve with yogurt mixed with 1-2 Tbsp. maple syrup.

Applesauce, Cooked

3 medium Apples pared,
cored and sliced
Add Honey or Brown Sugar to taste

Put apple slices in saucepan half covered with cold water. Boil until soft about 15 minutes. Put through food mill and mix with honey.

Applesauce, Fresh

3 medium Apples pared cored and sliced
Add Honey or Brown Sugar to taste

Run apples through the grinder portion of the juicer. Season to taste and enjoy.

Apple Spice Cake*

Combine:

1/4 Cup Honey or Maple Syrup
1 Cup fresh Applesauce
1 1/2 Cups Oat Flour
3/4 Cup Whole Wheat Flour or Triticale Flour

Sift together:

3/4 Cup Crude Brown Sugar
pinch Allspice
pinch Mace
1/4 tsp. Coriander
1 tsp. featherweight sodium free Baking Powder (optional)

Add:

2 Cups Raisins or chopped Dates

Combine wet and dry ingredients. Pour into non-stick oblong bake pan. Mix crumb topping and sprinkle on top. Bake at 325 degrees for 40 minutes or until cake tests done. Serve with a spoonful of fresh applesauce or nonfat yogurt. Enjoy.

*This is a potassium based baking powder. If you are a cancer patient, check with your physician first.

Crumb Topping

2/3 cup Rolled Oats
1/3 cup Maple Syrup or Honey
pinch Allspice
pinch Mace

Buzz oats briefly in blender to make a finer flake. Mix spices with oats. Mix in enough sweetener to make a crumbly mixture.

Apple Streusel Pie

1- 9" Pie Crust (see below)
12 med. Green Apples, sliced thin
1/3 cup crude Brown Sugar or 1/4 cup honey
2 tsp. Cornstarch or Oat Flour
2-3 tsp. Lemon or Orange Juice
1/2 cup Dried Currants or chopped Dates
pinch Coriander, Mace, Allspice

Combine dry ingredients. Coat apples. Drizzle on honey (if used) and juice. Fill pie crust. Sprinkle on topping. Bake at 300-325 F for 1 hr 15 min. or until apples are tender.

Crumb Topping

2/3 cup Oat Flour
3 tsp. Crude Brown Sugar
pinch Allspice
1/3 cup Honey or Maple Syrup

Apple-Sweet Potato Pudding

1 tsp. Raisins
*1/2 cup Bread Crumbs**
1/2 cup Orange Juice
1 Sweet Potato (boiled-peeled-sliced)
1 Apple (raw-peeled-sliced)
1 tsp. Brown Sugar

Place sweet potato slices in baking dish with apple slices and raisins spread with bread crumbs sugar and orange juice and bake in oven for 30 minutes. Serve hot with 3 tsp. buttermilk or yogurt if permitted.

***Note:** never use commercial bread crumbs (see recipe for bread crumbs in the bread section, pg. 100).

Apple Tart DAIRY, PG. 98

1/2 Cup warm water
(105-110 degrees F)
1 Tbsp. crude brown sugar (Sucanat)
1 package dry yeast
*2/3 Cup churned buttermilk, non-fat yogurt or apple juice**
1/2 Cup crude brown sugar (Sucanat)
2 1/2 Cups oat flour
1 Cup whole wheat or triticale flour
9-10 medium apples, gala, pippin or golden delicious are good
4 Tbsp. maple syrup, or liquid Fruit Source †
4 Tbsp. brown rice syrup †
1/2 Cup date sugar (dried ground dates)
1 1/2 tsp. allspice
1/4 tsp. mace or coriander
Use only apple juice if patient is not yet allowed dairy.

† Fruit Source is a sweetener derived from natural fruit sugars. Rice syrup, derived from malted rice, is a thick and creamy syrup that needs to be thinned by either the maple syrup or Fruit Source.

Sprinkle yeast onto warm water into which I tablespoon crude brown sugar has been dissolved. Let stand for 5 to 10 minutes or until frothy. Warm buttermilk, yogurt or juice to 100° F. Add crude brown sugar and stir until dissolved. Stir buttermilk into yeast mix, then add oat flour and beat vigorously. Stir in enough of the remaining flour to make a stiff dough. Knead on a floured bread board, adding only enough flour to keep dough from sticking. Knead until smooth and elastic, approximately 5 to 10 minutes. Place in a bowl, cover with tea towel and let rise in a warm place until double in bulk, about 1 1/2 hours. Punch down and let rise again.

Divide dough in half. On floured board, press each part into a 15" x 9" rectangle. Place on separate non-stick bake sheets, or regular sheets that have been thoroughly coated with oat flakes to prevent sticking. Prick surface with fork, leaving 1/4" border around the edges. Cover and let rise until doubled, approximately 40 minutes.

Quarter, core and slice apples, arranging each sliced quarter over dough, as you cut it. Place the flat side down and the skin side up, fanning the slices out slightly. Leave about a 1/2" border. Mix maple and brown rice syrups. Using a pastry brush, coat the apples with the syrup. Combine date sugar and spices and sprinkle over apples. Bake at 325° F. for 30 minutes or until bread is lightly browned. Serve as is or with a spoonful of non-fat yogurt or yogurt cheese (see note below) lightly sweetened with honey or maple syrup.

Note: *(Non-Gerson family members could enjoy this dessert with a scoop of non-fat fruit sweetened frozen yogurt - Cascadian Farm Vanilla (the milk is organic) or Stars Vanilla Bean are two brands I have enjoyed in moderation).*

* Yogurt cheese is made by draining non-fat yogurt through a stainless steel or nylon sieve lined with a cotton tea towel or cheese cloth with a bowl beneath to catch the whey. Refrigerate and drain until desired consistency is achieved, anywhere from 2 to 8 hours. A short drainage period will yield a thickened yogurt, longer periods will produce a cream cheese like texture. For our purposes, a thickened yogurt texture is what we want.

Apricots

1/2 lb. fresh Apricots
1 tsp. Cornstarch dissolved in 2 tsp. cold Water
2 tsp. Brown Sugar

Cut apricots in halves and remove pits. Place in pot with boiling water and cook for 10 minutes. Add cornstarch during last 2 minutes. Add sugar when cool.

Banana (Broiled)

1 Banana
1 Tsp. Brown sugar

Cut banana in half lengthwise add 1 tsp. brown sugar and few drops lemon. Place in pan and broil under low flame for 10 minutes. Serve hot.

Banana And Apple

1 banana (peeled and finely mashed)
1 apple (peeled-cored-grated)
10 tsp. raisins

Mix banana and apple beating thoroughly with fork or egg beater. Add raisins and serve.

Banana And Figs

1 banana
3 figs (fresh)
juice of 1 orange

Chop banana and figs fine and mix well with orange juice. Fill orange peel with this mixture and serve.

Cherries (Stewed)

1/2 lb. cherries (washed-stemmed)
1 tsp. potato starch
2 tsp. brown sugar

Place cherries in saucepan with water to cover cook 10 minutes over low flame add potato starch dissolved in 2 tsp. cold water. Add to boiling cherries. Cook 2 minutes longer. Chill and serve.

Currants

1/4 box red currants
3 tsp. brown sugar

Clean and wash currants thoroughly before removing stems. Place in dish add sugar and serve. Buttermilk or yogurt (if permitted) sweetened with brown sugar may be used for sauce.

Fruit Combination

3 cup fresh cherries and apricots (halved-sliced-pitted)
2 cup water
1/2 cup brown sugar
2 tsp. cornstarch dissolved in 1/3 cup cold water

Place fruit with water and sugar in saucepan. Boil gently slowly for 10 min. Add cornstarch. Cook 3 minutes longer. Cool and serve.

Glazed Pear Halves

4-5 Ripe Pears
4 Tbsp. Honey or Sucanat (organic dried cane sugar)

Cut ripe pears into halves, and core. Add about 4 oz. of water to honey or Sucanat and mix well. Place pear halves in baking dish and pour sugar mixture over fruit. Bake in slow oven (275 degrees F) until done. Baste with juice if necessary.

Frozen Yogurt +DAIRY, PG. 98

¼ cup stewed fruit (cherries, apricots are great)
1 lb. Fat-free yogurt

Spoon yogurt into a thin mesh strainer that has been lined with two layers of cheesecloth, and place it over a deep bowl. Let it drain into the bowl in the refrigerator for about 30 minutes. Spoon the drained yogurt into ice cube trays and freeze. Mix fruit and yogurt cubes into a food processor or the grinder of your K&K or Norwalk. The consistency is thick and smooth. Serve immediately.

Oatmeal Cake

4 cup Oatmeal (dry oats)
2 grated or blended Carrots
Honey and Raisins as desired

Combine all the above ingredients in a baking dish. Put in the oven without a lid and bake for 45 minutes at 250 degrees.

Oatmeal Cookies DAIRY, PG. 98

1 cup Apple Sauce
1 cup Rye Flour
1 cup Raisins
1/2 cup Buttermilk
1/2 cup Brown Sugar
1/2 cup Molasses
2 cup Oatmeal
1 pkg. Yeast

Mix and let stand 10 minutes. Drop from teaspoon and bake in moderate oven about 20 minutes.

Pasha* (Uncooked Cheese Cake) DAIRY, PG. 98

1/4 cup fresh orange juice, strained
*1/2 cup chopped dried fruit**
4 cup soft or medium curd cottage cheese
1/2 cup honey,
or 3/4 cup brown sugar
raisins, dates, papaya, peaches, prunes, etc.

Mix all ingredients. Pour batter into a strainer or colander lined with a clean cotton cloth (muslin). Cover with a plate to weight it down. Place in a bowl or pan and refrigerate for 5-10 hours or until dry and firm. Turn out onto a plate and slice. Good as is, or on a slice of Essene bread.

Peaches

1/2 lb. peaches (skinned)
2 tsp. brown sugar

Wash peaches. Place in boiling water 1/2 minute, drain and peel. Cut in halves. Remove pits and place in saucepan with boiling water. Cover. Simmer for 10 minutes. Cool. Add sugar and serve chilled.

Pears

1 large pear (peeled-cored-cut in 1/2)
1 tsp. brown sugar

Place pears in saucepan with water to half cover. Add sugar and cook 30 min.

Plums

1/2 lb. plums
2 tsp. brown sugar

Wash plums, cut in halves and remove pits (Plums can also be cooked whole). Place in saucepan with water to cover. Cook 15 min. Remove, cool and add sugar. Serve chilled.

Prune And Apricots (Dried)

1/2 lb. of each
1/3 cup barley

Soak prunes and apricots over night in water to cover. Use same water and boil with barley. Cool and serve.

Prune and Banana Whip

1 cup dried prunes (soaked-cooked)
2 small bananas
1/4 lemon juice
1 tsp. brown sugar

Whip together thoroughly and put in refrigerator for 1 hour. May be served in slices decorated with sweetened yogurt (if permitted)

Pumpkin Pudding Pie* (Unbaked)

pinch Allspice
pinch Coriander
pinch Mace
2 tsp. unsulphered Molasses (optional)
1- 8" or 9" Pie Crust
1/2 cup Tapioca
1 1/2 cup Dates, pitted and chopped
1 1/3 cup Apple Juice or Water
1 1/2 to 2 cup mashed Pumpkin

Soak tapioca and dates in juice overnight. In morning stew over low flame using a burner pad to diffuse heat. Cook for 30 minutes stirring frequently to prevent sticking. This will be very thick. Puree tapioca and pumpkin in Foley food mill or processor. Add spices and molasses. Pour into prepared pie crust and chill thoroughly (may put in freezer for several hours until very firm), otherwise cutting will be a problem. Serve with a dollop of honey sweetened yogurt cheese* if desired (and permitted by physician).

Variation
Use cooked squash, yams, or sweet potatoes in place of pumpkin.

Thin Buttermilk Crust DAIRY, PG. 98

1 & 1/4 cup oat flour
1/3 cup churned buttermilk, apple juice, or water (cold)
2 tsp. honey
pinch allspice or mace
1 tsp. Featherweight (sodium free) baking powder (optional)*

Mix dry ingredients. Add honey and just enough liquid to make a stiff dough. Knead lightly to mix. Roll out on floured board or between layers of waxed paper. Carefully place in pie plate which has been thoroughly coated with oat flakes to prevent sticking. Trim excess dough and flute edges or make indentations with fork. Chill crust, then bake at 325 degrees for 10-15 minutes or until lightly browned.

Note: This will not be your traditional flaky crust, so roll out thin.

Raised Crust*

1 Cup Oat Flour
1/2 Cup Potato Flour
(or use more oat flour)
1 Cup Triticale
or Whole Wheat Flour
1 tsp. Honey or Brown Sugar
1/2 Cup Warm Water
1 tsp. Baker's Yeast

Sprinkle yeast into warm water mixed with honey. When frothy add flour and mix well. Let rise in a warm place for 1 hour. Knead on floured board for 5 min. Let rest for 10 min., roll out on floured board. Place in pie plate that has been thoroughly coated on the bottom with rolled oat flakes. Flute edge. Let rise for 15 min. Bake at 375 F. for 20-25 min.

Variation

Omit yeast, use just enough cold water to make a stiff dough. Roll out between sheets of floured wax paper. Carefully place in pie plate. Chill crust. Then bake at 350 F for 10-12 min.

Essene Bread Crust*

2 Cup Essene Bread Crumbs
1/4 Cup Honey
3 tsp. Oat Flour

Toast slices of bread in slow oven until lightly brown. Let cool. Grind coarsely by running through grinder or Norwalk. Add flour, then honey. Press into pie plate that has been well coated with rolled oat flakes. Chill for 1 hour. Bake at 350 F for 10-12 min. Roll, then fill.

Rhubarb

1/2 lb. rhubarb (washed and cut into 1 inch pieces)
2 to 3 tsp. brown sugar (to taste)
1 tsp. cornstarch (if desired)

Place washed rhubarb in saucepan. Simmer 15 to 20 minutes. Dissolve cornstarch in a little cold water. Add to rhubarb and allow to stew a few more minutes. Cool and add sugar, (note: combine rhubarb with other sweet fruits such as apples-peaches-apricots (fresh or dried).

Stewed Fruit Combinations

pears and plums
plums and applesauce
peaches and plums
apricots and plums
apricots and sliced apples
peaches and pears

***note:** Stewed fruits may be served on toasted rye bread placing a thick layer of fruit - allowing it to soak through for 1/2 hour before serving.*

Sunshine Smoothie†

In a blender or food processor container, combine one cup non-fat organic yogurt, ½ cup orange juice , 2 tablespoons honey, 1 cup cut-up fresh fruit and ½ cup crushed ice (made from distilled water); process until smooth.

Sweet Potato and Apple Bake[GSG]

12 oz. sweet potatoes
3 eating apples
allspice
a little brown sugar
a little water

Cook the sweet potatoes gently in their skins until tender. Allow to cool. Slice and put into baking dish with alternative layers of apple. Over each layer, sprinkle some water, a little sugar and some allspice. Bake covered for 20 minutes at 350 degrees F, then remove cover and bake for an additional 10 minutes.

Sweet Potato Stuffed Oranges

3 lbs. Sweet Potatoes (or Yams)
Freshly made Apple Sauce
8 Orange peel halves
4 oz. orange juice

Boil sweet potatoes (or yams) until done. Peel and mash with orange juice and apple sauce to make it a smooth, stuffing paste. Put stuffing into orange peel halves and put a dab of apple sauce on top. Can be reheated in a cake tray. Makes 4 servings. Recipe may actually stuff 10 or more orange peels and may make more than 4 servings.)

Sweet Rice[MZ]

1 1/2 Cups organic brown rice
4 Cups water
1 Cup organic brown sugar (Sucanat)
1 Cup organic raisins

Wash the rice and put into pot with the water. Once the water begins to boil, add the sugar and raisins and reduce the heat. Maintain on low heat until the rice is tender.

Dairy

Dairy is temporarily forbidden in the beginning of therapy. Consult with your physician before adding any dairy to your diet.

After 6 to 12 weeks on the therapy, upon doctor's orders, animal proteins are cautiously added to the diet in the form of pot cheese, yogurt and cottage cheese, and churned (not cultured) buttermilk, all made from non-fat milk (preferably raw) and without salt.

When starting the proteins, it must be done slowly and carefully. Just one tablespoon at lunch and supper of the solid proteins and one-half cup of the buttermilk per meal. After 3-4 days, these levels can be increased until, at three weeks, one cup of solid dairy and one cup of yogurt or buttermilk per meal.

While adding the dairy proteins, the patient needs to watch for signs that the body is tolerating the new foods. Indigestion, flatulence (intestinal production of gas) and nasal mucus production are signs the enzyme activity cannot yet handle the dairy products. The patient should reduce or, after consulting the physician, eliminate the proteins for several more weeks.

Yogurt DAIRY, SEE HEADING

Combine:

2 quarts raw non-fat milk
(heated to 118 F)
1 pkg. "Bulgarian Yogurt Culture"
or 3 tsp. yogurt (purchased
or saved from a previous batch)

Pour mixture into sterilized glass jar(s). Incubate between 110-115 F for 4-8 hours by one of the following methods:

*Electric yogurt maker
*In gas oven, above pilot light
*In electric oven, low heat (gauge heat with thermometer)
*In a thermos
*In a covered pan set in a container of warm water (change water to keep warm)

Incubation time may vary, depending upon temperature. Ready when a toothpick inserted point first into the yogurt doesn't fall over. The yogurt becomes set a little more firmly after refrigeration. But this is a thin yogurt because it has no fat and processed dried milk added. Be sure to save 3 Tbsp. for the starter for the next batch.

Yogurt Cheese DAIRY, SEE HEADING

Yogurt cheese is made by hanging non-fat yogurt in a muslin sack over a sink or bowl or in a muslin lined strainer until it thickens to the consistency of cream cheese - without the fat - in about 6 to 8 hours.

Cottage Cheese Loaf*

DAIRY, SEE HEADING

1 cup dry Essene
or rye bread crumbs
1 tbsp. lemon juice or vinegar
1-2 tsp. dried parsley
1/2 tsp. dillweed or tarragon
1/2 tsp. dry horseradish
(1 tsp. if fresh)
2 cups mashed potatoes
2-1/3 cups dry curd cottage cheese
1/2 cup sweet red or green pepper
1/2 cup celery, diced
1 small onion, diced

Combine all ingredients except the last two. Form into a loaf. Place on garnished platter. Top with decorative veggie slices. watercress or endive for garnish, slices of carrot, tomato, onion, green or red pepper for top.

Cottage Cheese DAIRY, SEE HEADING

by Yvonne Nienstadt

1/2 gallon raw, non-fat milk, (unopened - May not be available)

Makes approx. 9 oz. (1 cup) cheese. Warm milk to body temperature (98-100 °F) by placing unopened bottle in sink of warm water. Incubate in warm place (near pilot light or in oven with light on). It is best to leave milk in original container to prevent airborne bacteria or molds from contaminating culture. The incubation period is about 24-30 hours. (Culture longer for a sharper cheese) Shake several times during this period.

When curd has formed, it will rise to the top. A harder curd can be formed by putting cheese (still in bottle) in sink of warm water and gradually increasing temperature to 110° for soft curd, and to 120° for farmer style cheese. Be careful not to overheat or you will destroy precious enzymes and beneficial bacteria. Use a thermometer to be safe.

Pour cheese into a strainer or colander lined with muslin or several layers of cheese cloth. Gather the corners of the cloth and press out whey. You may place a weight on top to speed the process.

For 'cream' style cottage cheese add approx. 1/4 cup thick yogurt per cup of finished cheese.

For 'herbed' cottage cheese, season with any of the following: fresh chives, crushed garlic, tarragon. parsley, dill weed. dill seed. Let set for 1/2 hr. before serving.

Variations

Add the juice of 1 or 2 lemons or 1/8 Cup yogurt to the fresh milk instead of letting it clabber naturally. These additions result in different flavors and textures. Experiment to find the one you like the best. Enjoy!

Cottage Cheese Sour Cream*DAIRY, SEE HEADING

1/2 cup yogurt
1 Tbsp. lemon juice
1 Cup dry curd cottage cheese

Blend ingredients in blender. Add any or all of the following: Pressed garlic, grated horseradish, chives or green onion, fresh mint or dried dill weed. Use to top baked potatoes or as dip for veggies.

Breads

Bread can be used as a snack, after breakfast, or with a meal if the patient has a good appetite. Do not replace potatoes and vegetables with bread.

Sourdough

Sourdough is sour fermented dough used as leaven. Don't be put off by the name - sourdough breads don't taste sour. They have a tangy flavor. Sourdough is a white substance over which a colorless or gray liquor called hooch collects. Hooch enables sourdough to complete its fermentation You have to feed sourdough and keep it in the refrigerator because it is a living thing - full of microorganisms. Colonies of these microorganisms can live for many decades with proper care and feeding. You can use a starter batch obtained from someone else to get your own going or buy a dehydrated starter or make it from scratch. There are many different kinds of sourdough starters: white - yogurt - whole wheat - sour rye - etc. For patients on the Gerson Therapy Rye Sourdough is the recommended variety.

Sourdough Starter

1 tsp. Active Dry Yeast
3 cup warm Water
(105-115 degrees F)
3-1/2 cups Rye Flour

1. Dissolve yeast in warm water in a large mixing bowl. Set aside for about 5 minutes.

2. Gradually add flour stirring until smooth with a wooden spoon.

3. Cover with cheesecloth: leave on counter in warm draft-free place. in about 24 hours the mixture will start to ferment.

4. Cover tightly with plastic wrap and leave for another 2 to 3 days. Stir starter 2 or 3 times a day.

5. Starter should be foamy at the end of this time. Put into a plastic container- glass jar - or crock with at least a 1-quart capacity. Stir - cover - but not with tight-fitting top.

Feeding Sourdough

Put 1 cup sourdough in mixing bowl. Add 2 and 1/2 cups flour and 2 cups warm water. (this is known as feeding.) Mix thoroughly. Leave on counter for 8 hours or overnight. Be sure to replace 1 c sourdough in the jar in the refrigerator. Try to feed sourdough once a week or every 10 days. Feeding is necessary to keep it alive and may add tang to the flavor (note: sourdough can be frozen).

General Rules Pertaining To Sourdough

*Use glass, stoneware, or plastic bowls. Don't use metal. Wild yeast produces acids that can corrode metal and thus kill the starter.
*Use a wooden spoon
*Clean container about every week so that unwanted bacteria will not grow and ruin your sourdough.
*Wipe up spilled sourdough immediately. It can stick like glue or cement.
*Keep covered with a loose-fitting cover in refrigerator.

Wholegrain Rye bread

6 cups lukewarm Water
Sourdough Starter
3 lbs. Rye Flour or 70/30 Rye

and Whole Wheat Flour

Mix sourdough in water, add flour. Leave covered and warm (180 degrees) for 12-24 hours. Replace 1 cup sourdough to refrigerator as starter for next time.

Add:

2 cups lukewarm Water
2 lbs. rinsed Whole Rye Grain
2 Lbs. Rolled Rye
(enough Rye Flour (maybe 2 Lbs.) to hold dough together)

Roll and cut dough to fit loaf pans, smooth the surface with a wet hand and leave in a warm place to rise for 2-5 hours. The taste gets stronger the longer it is left to rise and it will rise only a little. Cut a furrow down the middle and this should be about 1/4 to 1/2 inch deep.

Bake for 1 and 1/2 hours at 385 degrees. Take out of pans immediately and wrap in towels and turn upside down. Do not cut for about 12 hours, bread can be frozen when lukewarm.

Bread Snack

1 slice of bread, spread with cottage cheese, topped with tomatoes, and radishes or sprouts or 1 slice of bread topped with honey.

Bread Dressing

1 part Chopped Onions
1 part Chopped Celery
2-3 parts cubed Grain Bread
1/2 part chopped Parsley
1/2 to 1 cup water
Sage, Garlic, Thyme

Place in an uncovered casserole and bake in low oven 2 hours,

Bread Crumbs

Toast leftover bread in the oven. Run through the food grinder. Store in covered container in the refrigerator.

Sour Rye Bread (Black Bread Russian Style)

Note; *Sour Rye is a different sourdough culture. You will need to make the sour rye sourdough starter from scratch and keep it separate from your other starter.*

8 Cups freshly ground Whole Rye Flour
3 Cups warm Water
1/2 Cup Sourdough Culture

Mix seven cups of the rye flour with water and sourdough culture. Cover and let stand in a warm place 12 to 18 hours. (Remove and save 1/2 cup of dough as a culture for next baking. Keep the culture in a tightly closed jar in refrigerator.) Add remaining cup of rye flour and mix well. Divide dough in half. Form oblong loaf smaller than size of pan in lightly floured hands (using rye flour).

Place gently into stainless steel baking pans. Do not press: allow space around sides of loaf.

Try dusting stainless steel pan with flour or rye meal, no oil. Let rise for approximately one half-hour. Bake at 350 degrees F. for one hour or more. Makes 2 two-pound loaves. Store tightly wrapped in refrigerator.

Sourdough Culture

In wide mouthed glass jar at least one quart in size Mix well the following ingredients:

1 cup lukewarm Distilled Water
2 tsp. Baking Yeast
1 tsp. Raw Sugar
1 cup Rye Flour

Stir well once daily with a wooden spoon (never leave a metal spoon in starter).* Allow to sit for 3 to 5 days until sour odor is detected* May cover LOOSELY after 2nd day Remove one-half cup for bread recipe above* Store covered in refrigerator adding half cup from dough after first rising. Bring to room temperature one hour before starting each new recipe

Sourdough Potato Rye Bread*

1 Cup Sourdough Starter
2 Cups warm Mashed Potatoes
1-1/3 Cups Potato Cooking Water
*2 Cups Whole Wheat or Rye Flour**
1/4 Cup Molasses (unsulphured)
1/3 tsp. Caraway or Fennel Seed

Mix ingredients in large non-metal bowl. Cover and let stand in warm place for several hours (or overnight for a very sour loaf). Add the following:

1-1/2 to 3 cup Rye Flour as needed to make a workable dough

Turn on to floured board and knead for 5-10 minutes. Let dough rest for 5 minutes, then form into round or baton shaped loaves. Place on Teflon or regular bake sheet (ungreased) that has been well coated with raw oat flakes to prevent sticking. Let bread rise until almost double (when bread does not spring back when lightly touched). Bake at 350 degrees for 50 minutes to 1 hour. For a very chewy crust, place a pan of water in bottom of oven to create steam, or baste bread several times during baking with water. For soft crust, do not steam or baste. Immediately wrap loaves in cotton towels upon leaving oven. Let bread cool before cutting.

* Dr. Gerson allowed patients to use 1/3 wheat to 2/3 rye flour. The bread is delicious with or without wheat.

Sourdough Squash Rye Bread

1 Cup Sourdough Starter
2 Cups Pureed Cooked Squash

(such as Butternut or Kabocha)
1 1/3 Cups Water
2 Cups Rye Flour
1/4 Cup Honey
1/4 Cup Potato Flour

Mix dry ingredients in ceramic or plastic bowl. Cover and let stand in warm place to proof (85 to 95 is ideal.) Add 2 cups rye flour, then 1 1/2 to 3 cups more rye flour until achieving workable dough. Turn into floured board and knead for 5-10 minutes. Let dough rest for 5 minutes, then shape into loaves or rolls. Sprinkle bottom of baking pans with raw oats, then let rise for 2 hours or until doubled in size. Bake at 350 for an hour. Let loaves cool before slicing.

Carrot Raisin Quick Bread*

1-1/2 cups Triticale or Rye Flour
1-1/2 cups Brown Rice or Oat Flour
1 cup Whole Wheat or Rye Flour
5 cups Carrots, grated
*2-1/2 cups Orange Pulp**
1/3-1/2 cups Honey
2 cups Raisins
1/2 tsp. each Allspice & Coriander
** approx. 2 large Navels, peeled and ground*

Sift dry ingredients together. Stir in raisins. Mix the remaining ingredients, then gradually stir into dry mix. Dough should be rather firm. Divide in half and fill two non-stick bake pans. Bake at 325 degrees for 50 minutes or until toothpick comes out clean. Let cool before removing from pan.

Essene Bread*

This naturally sweet cakey bread is made with only sprouted grain. The original recipe comes from The Essene Gospel of Peace, a 2,000 year old Aramaic text, which reveals the process of sprouting wheat as follows: "Moisten your wheat, that the angel of water may enter it. Then set it in the air, that the angel of air may also embrace it. And leave it from morning to evening beneath the sun, that the angel of sunshine may descend upon it."

This modern version differs from the original only in the use of oven heat instead of the sun's.

For one loaf use: 1 quart of 2 day old wheat, rye, or triticale sprouts.

Refrigerate sprouts for one day, uncovered, to dry slightly. Do not rinse before grinding or you will wind up with more of a pudding than bread.

Grind in hand or electric grinder or in the Norwalk using the #2 grid (second to the largest). Feed sprouts gradually or they will set up like cement in your grinding mechanism.

Shape into 1 1/2" to 2" high loaf. Place on non-stick or regular baking sheet well coated with oat flakes to prevent sticking. Bake at 250-300 degrees for 1 1/2 to 2 1/2 hours (loaf should be nicely browned). Cool thoroughly before slicing (chilled is best). Use serrated knife with a gently sawing motion. It also helps to dip knife in cold water before slicing bread.

Variations

Fruit Bread

Add:

1/3 or 2/3 cup raisins or other chopped dried fruit
1/2 tsp. coriander, mace, or allspice.

Onion or Garlic Herb Bread

Add:

2 or 3 Tbsp. finely minced onion, or 2-4 cloves pressed garlic
1/2 to 1 tsp. dill, thyme, caraway or fennel.

Wafers or Crackers

Form into 1/4" patties or roll out on floured board and cut into squares. Bake on non-stick or oat coated baking sheet at 250-300 degrees for 45 min. to 1 hour.

Appendix IV: Adapting the Gerson Therapy for Chemo-pre-treated Patients

Dr. Gerson's book, *A Cancer Therapy - Results of 50 Cases* does not mention chemotherapy anywhere. The reason is that during the time he practiced, chemo was just being researched and rarely used. An exception is the case of Johnny Gunther (Appendix II, p. 415) who had been treated with one of the first experimental drugs. At the time of Johnny's death, Dr. Gerson was devastated because he truly loved the boy. He took the blame for his death and felt it was due to the hormone treatment he had permitted to be used. As we have found out in the meantime, the hormones could have contributed to the damage; but the boy exhibited what we now recognize as a typical "6th month chemo flare-up". Since this was the very first chemo case Dr. Gerson was treating, he didn't realize the specific changes that take place under those circumstances..

In our 22 years of experience using the Gerson Therapy under present conditions, we have understandably run across a fair percentage of patients pre-treated with now dozens of different "cytotoxic" (tissue-poisoning) drugs.

The first chemo-treated patients that were accepted for treatment at the Mexican Gerson Hospital at approximately the same time were suffering from breast cancer. It was assumed that it would be wise to 'detoxify' these patients as thoroughly as possible to remove the administered poisons. Therefore the physicians administered the castor oil treatment (commonly used in Gerson patients) to those patients as well. The shock came when the physicians observed that the castor oil tended to remove those toxins too rapidly releasing them into the blood stream and actually causing these patients to suffer from an overdose of chemo. These 2 patients had to be transferred to intensive care! In other words, it became evident that chemo-treated patients must be treated cautiously and detoxified slowly.

In the meantime, we have seen many such patients and a number of satisfactory long term recoveries have been recorded. (See one case in the *Gerson Healing Newsletter*, May/June 1999; Vol. 14, #3).

We give below the suggested modifications of the basic Gerson Therapy as described in *A Cancer Therapy: Results of Fifty Cases*, by Dr. Max Gerson. Naturally, the exact treatment, number of juices, enemas, medications etc. are adjusted by a Gerson trained physician; but this is the basic daily protocol.

Basic Daily Protocol for the Modified Therapy:

- 13 glasses of 8 oz. each of a variety of juices (apple/carrot, carrot green, orange)
  Reduced in severely damaged patients to 8 glasses; or thirteen 4-6 oz. glasses
- 20 teaspoons of potassium compound (2 tsp. In each of 10 glasses)
- 1 1/2 tp 3 grains thyroid
- 6 drops 1/2 strength Lugol's solution
- 6 tablets of 50 mg. Niacin (omit if bleeding is present)
- 6 capsules Acidol Pepsin
- 12 tablets Pancreatin
- 6 Dessicated Liver Capsules
- 3 cc liver extract with 50 mcg B-12 (1 intramuscular injection daily)
- 3 coffee enemas
- CoQ-10 - -Begin at 60 mg the first day, if no side effects are observed, increase dosage to 300 mg. per day, then 600 mg on the third day and thereafter.
- 2 g (2,000 mg) Vitamin C (Ascorbic Acid)

- The diet is unchanged, and includes 2 tablespoonfuls of organic flax seed oil daily.
  See Table on Page 3

Caster Oil Enemas are Omitted from the Modified Therapy!

Appendix V: A Gerson Patient's Problems - How to Avoid Mistakes

By Charlotte Gerson

It has frequently occurred to me that, in order to really be sure that the patients understand and follow the Gerson Therapy exactly, I ought to follow them around their house and kitchen for 24 hours. The situation that occurred last week-end amply illustrates the point. I was surprised and shocked because I certainly didn't expect to find the following situation. But since it was taking place I feel that I need to share my concerns with our friends and other patients in order to make them aware and prevent errors.

The patient in question was not only very much interested in the Gerson Therapy for his own recovery but he feels so strongly about spreading the word of healing that he organized a Gerson Convention Day. He also invited me to stay at his lovely home overnight so that I could be spoiled with good, organic Gerson food and juices.

The house is located in a wooded area, with beautiful huge trees, and at the edge of a small lake. In other words, the air is clean and fresh and the atmosphere relaxing - no problem there. The patient's business is well organized and runs quite well with minimal attention, so he is able to get a lot of rest. There is help in the household, so there are no pressures in the juice and food preparation. But there are at least four major problems in the patient's application of the Therapy:

1. The water is 'hard'; it contains minerals. So, like other people in the area, the patient's home is equipped with "water softener' equipment. His very warm, concerned and cooperative wife is doing everything in her power to help her husband recover. Yet she stated that she brings in "sacks of salt" for the water softener! As our readers know, in the process of removing the unwelcome minerals in the water, the equipment replaces these with sodium. What happens as a result is that the patient washes and bathes in "softened water", loaded with salt. Salt is very easily absorbed through the skin and should never be used by a Gerson patient. Salt is an enzyme inhibitor and the Gerson Therapy is designed to remove all excess of sodium. Salt is needed for fast growth of tumor tissue. It is also the basis of the "tissue damage syndrome", when normal cells lose their ability to hold potassium while sodium penetrates, causing edema and loss of function. This tissue damage is, according to Dr. Gerson, the beginning of all chronic disease. Naturally, bathing in salt water must be avoided at all cost.

2. We were served a very delicious and attractive lunch which included a lovely salad loaded with avocados. I immediately asked if the patient, too, was eating them. He was! That is another serious mistake, since avocados contain a fairly large percentage of fat. This is the reason why they are forbidden, because fats tend to stimulate new tumor growth! The lady of the house said that she thought that avocados were served at Meridien - which they are not. The problem here is that the patient or caregiver should not rely on memory. All these items are clearly set down in the *A Cancer Therapy*; and avocados are the second item on the Forbidden list. We have to ask patients and caregivers to read and re-read the "Therapy" Chapter in the book, Chapter XXXIII, p. 237, and make sure that they understand all the directions exactly and follow all instructions.

3. Along with the lunch, we had a very nice vegetable soup. It contained some zucchini, peas, celery and onions and a few other vegetables. The patient asked me how I enjoyed the "Hippocrates Soup". I had to state that the soup we had was not Hippocrates soup, as Dr. Gerson describes it in the book. The combination of ingredients that are supposed to be in that soup are clearly described in the book as well as in this book, the *Gerson Therapy Handbook* and are very specific. Actually, Hippocrates (the father of medicine) already understood that this

special combination of ingredients has a beneficial, detoxifying effect on the kidneys. That is the reason why Dr. Gerson used it. He felt that this soup was so important that he wanted patients to eat this 'special soup' twice daily to benefic the kidneys and help them to clear toxins from the body. Occasionally, one can add some extra tomatoes, in season, to give the soup a different flavor; or one can cut up and roast some onions on a dry cookie sheet (NO fat, butter or oil) in the oven. Then these can be added to the same basic soup recipe for a taste treat. However, the basic recipe remains unchanged,

4. The lady of the house also thoughtfully offered me some enema coffee which I gladly accepted. When I picked it up for use, however, I seriously wondered whether it was the proper strength. I have used enemas for many years and know pretty well what the coffee should look like. This solution seemed too weak to be considered, "concentrate" for dilution 4 to 1. The lady 'thought' that she used the recipe in the *Handbook* and that it was right. The caregiver must be sure that each enema contains the equivalent of 3 rounded tablespoons of coffee (See *A Cancer Therapy*, p.247). If a concentrate is prepared, each portion MUST contain the 3 tablespoons of coffee. The coffee enema, too, is so very important that it is imperative that the mixture or solution is correct. Please check and recheck the preparation of the coffee concentrate.

5. Somewhat less important than the above 4 points: The patient enjoys some bread with his meals - which is quite acceptable. But it is also important to understand that the main needs for nutrition are the salads, soup, potato and vegetables, and fruit. If all those foods have been consumed, it is alright for the patient to also have a slice of unsalted rye bread. Bread should never be the main part of a meal.

Unfortunately, in the last few months, we have had several patients who failed. I also discussed this problem with the most experienced Gerson Therapy doctors: Alicia Melendez and Luz Maria Bravo. Aside from the above, there are other problems we have run across. Let me state here that we (the Gerson doctors as well as myself when I talk to patients) have a serious problem. When we ask the patient about their compliance with the Gerson Therapy directives, even the above patient who made serious errors, will assure us that he is doing everything 'perfectly'. These patients don't realize what is wrong with their version of the Therapy.

When we try to help, heal, and direct the patient to the Gerson Therapy, we rely on the various tools that we have specially created to give the patient and family every possible help and guidance: the food preparation video-tape and the recipe book in the *Handbook*; the 4-hour workshop tape discussing in detail as much of the treatment as we can and, most important, Dr. Gerson's book. At this point, I need to stress again that the patient must familiarize himself very thoroughly with this material and review it over and over again.

One problem area that keeps coming up is the food preparation. Just boiling the food and putting it on the plate is not good enough. The food preparation tape initiates the cook into various areas to make foods tasty. For example, cooked beets when pealed and sliced can be reheated a little with some freshly made apple sauce, stirred, and the vegetable then resembles "Harvard beets". Or, the sliced beets can be dressed with onions, some green pepper strips and vinegar with flax-seed oil dressing for a beet salad. During the summer months, these salads (also potato salad, string bean or butter bean salad, etc.) are very welcome, refreshing and appetite stimulators. There are many suggested recipes in the back of the *Handbook* that, I am afraid, are being disregarded. As a result, we get the report that the patient is weak, is losing weight, and is doing poorly. Almost always, it turns out that they have 'cravings' for pizza, enchilada, or some other greasy, salty, forbidden food. They are simply hungry because they are not eating the healing, nutritious Gerson meals which are not well prepared.

The Gerson food has another advantage: if the patient (or family member for that matter) eats fresh, organic food, it is truly satisfying and we often get reports that the companions lose their cravings for sweets or heavy desserts. But the key is tasty food that is prepared with imagination and inspiration from the recipes provided. I must remind, patients frequently that when they are on a nutritional therapy, they are on nothing if they don't eat! If patients eat properly, we have seen most gain weight if they are emaciated. Some who are too heavy will lose weight on the same regimen.

The summer fruit are especially valuable, high in potassium enzymes and the best nutrients: cherries, apricots, peaches, nectarines, plums, pears, grapes and more. But not far behind are apples that are available virtually all year round. Patients (unless they are diabetic or suffer from Candida) should always eat much fruit at night, first thing in the morning, and anytime between meals. One summer food presents a problem: corn. It is perfectly alright to eat corn. The difficulty is that everybody loves corn and during the season is likely to eat it to the exclusion of other vegetables. That is a very bad idea. The vegetables should provide variety and a large selection of special healing chemicals (phytochemicals) and trace minerals. Eating mostly one vegetable is not acceptable and does not fulfill the purpose.

Let the guiding spirit of the patient be: "I'll do the best possible to help my sick body heal" rather than "I'll see how little I can do and still get away with it".